School Start – **Access your onli...e resources**

School Start is accompanied by a number of printable online materials, designed to ensure this resource best supports your professional needs.

Activate your accompanying online resources
- Go to www.routledge.com/cw/speechmark then click on the cover of this book
- Click the 'Sign in or Request Access' button and follow the instructions, in order to access your accompanying online resources

SCHOOL START

SECOND EDITION

Targeted intervention for Language and
Sound Awareness in reception class

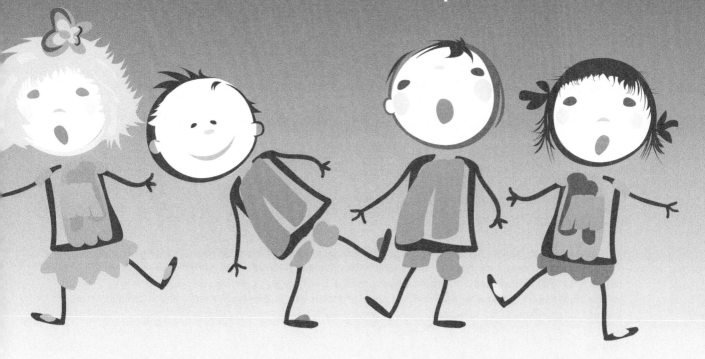

Catherine de la Bedoyere and Catharine Lowry

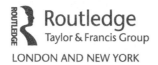 Routledge
Taylor & Francis Group

LONDON AND NEW YORK

First published 2015 by Speechmark Publishing Ltd.

Published 2017 by Routledge
2 Park Square, Milton Park, Abingdon, Oxon OX14 4RN
711 Third Avenue, New York, NY 10017, USA

Routledge is an imprint of the Taylor & Francis Group, an informa business

British Library Cataloguing in Publication Data
A catalogue record for this book is available from the British Library

ISBN 9781909301580 (pbk)

Contents

Preface to the second edition   iv

Preface to the first edition   v

Acknowledgements   vi

Part 1 Introduction   **1**

How to use this resource   3

Sample Group Session Sheets   13

Using the *School Start* website   19

Part 2 Group Session Sheets   **21**

Language Sessions 1–30   23

Sound Awareness Sessions 1–30   55

Part 3 Resource Templates   **87**

List of Resource Templates   88

Language Templates 1–44   91

Sound Awareness Templates 45–70   137

Part 4 Programme Delivery Templates   **165**

Record Sheets   167

Starting the programme   181

Handouts for home and class   191

Bibliography   207

Preface to the second edition

We are delighted to present the second edition of our programme *School Start*. Since its first publication it has been warmly received across the UK and is now in place in many schools. In some locations it is adopted by every infant or primary school in that local authority. Many schools have now been using this resource for over 10 years. Further evidence to support the value and effectiveness of this intervention comes from a study by the authors based in Brighton and Hove and through an independent study in South Ribble.

This second edition retains the session plans and their activities and resources. User feedback suggested that we clarify some aspects of help with how to deliver the programme, for example elaborating on how to use the checklists. We have also emphasised and simplified how to transfer skills learned within the group into the home and classroom.

Changes in special educational needs are reflected in how we refer to the programme as a 'targeted' intervention that derives from Marie Gascoigne's model of The Balanced System (Gascoigne, 2015) and how this intervention may form part of a child's Educational, Health and Care Plan (UK, Government, 2014a).

Changes in technology mean that the resources associated with the *School Start* programme are now available on the website at www.routledge.com/cw/speechmark

Catherine de la Bedoyere and Catharine Lowry
July 2015

Authors' note

Please note that, for the sake of simplicity alone, the masculine pronoun 'he' is used in the activity descriptions to refer to the individual child and the feminine pronoun 'she' is used to refer to the teaching assistant or reception class teacher.

For readers outside the UK, the age ranges for the classes mentioned are as follows: Reception year (4–5 years) and Year 1 (5–6 years).

Preface to the first edition

Teachers are becoming increasingly concerned about the communication skills of children entering school in the Reception year (4–5 years). In recent years there has been a focus of resources upon building skills in early years to prevent detrimental consequences for later learning and socialising. *Every Child Matters* (DfES, 2004) has pulled together society's aims for our youngsters, and schools are being asked to plan provision for the vulnerable children by providing in-class additional group support (Wave 2) and specific targeted approaches for children identified as requiring Special Educational Needs support (Wave 3). *School Start* is a programme that schools can use in the Reception year to raise the communication skills of their most vulnerable children.

Although reference has been made to the National Curriculum of England and Wales, the activities are not dependent on knowledge or experience of the National Curriculum and can be carried out by any English-speaking user.

School Start is:

- a programme comprising 30 group sessions for developing Language skills in reception class children
- a programme with 30 further group sessions for developing Sound Awareness skills in reception class children
- a programme that can be delivered by teaching assistants
- designed to be a preventive Wave 2 approach to developing delayed communication skills
- based on checklist assessment to identify target children and evaluate outcomes
- based on the Foundation Stage Curriculum.

School Start first began as a programme of group interventions written by speech and language therapists working in an infant language unit attached to a mainstream school. The programme was then extended for use by teaching assistants working with children in mainstream schools. It has been trialled and evaluated for three years across the Royal Borough of Kingston upon Thames. Each year it has been revised and simplified so that teaching assistants and schools feel confident to use the programme. Outcome measures have consistently demonstrated that children benefit from inclusion in the programme (see Figure 1). Schools have testified to its success by choosing to repeat the programme for successive intakes of children.

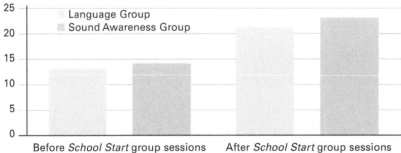

Figure 1: Mean scores before and after the implementation of *School Start* during trialling (Royal Borough of Kingston upon Thames, 2004/5)

Catherine de la Bedoyere and Catharine Lowry
February 2007

Acknowledgements

The authors would like to thank the staff in the schools, speech and language therapy departments and local authorities who have played an important part in developing this resource and are committed to offering this provision in all of the reception classes in their area.

In particular, we would like to recognise the contributions of the Royal Borough of Kingston upon Thames, Brighton and Hove and South Ribble.

Part 1
Introduction

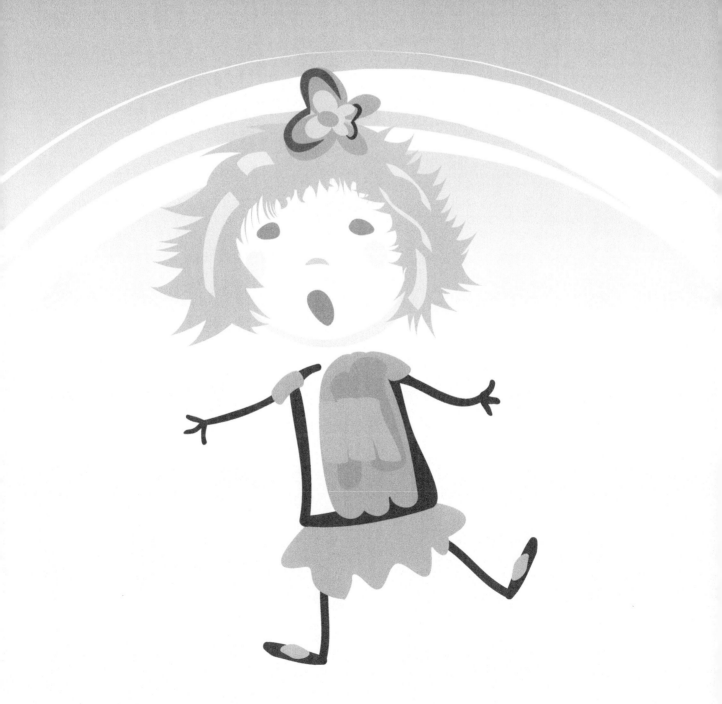

How to use this resource

This book is divided into four parts as follows.

Part 1 Introduction

Part 1 provides information on how to deliver the *School Start* programme. This information is designed to be used by:

- a school
- a school together with its local speech and language therapy department
- a children's trust or local authority wanting to promote *School Start* in all of its schools.

Part 2 Group Session Sheets

Part 2 contains all of the Group Session Sheets needed in order to deliver the programme (also available at www.routledge.com/cw/speechmark).

Part 3 Resource Templates

Part 3 contains the Resource Templates for Language and Sound Awareness referred to in the Group Session Sheets. All templates are provided in black and white, so that they may be easily photocopied. The accompanying website also provides the option to print some of the templates in colour. There is a full list of the templates that are available in colour in the List of Resource Templates in Part 3 (pages 88–9).

Part 4 Programme Delivery Templates

Part 4 contains all of the checklists, record sheets and handouts that you will need when delivering the programme. These can either be photocopied or downloaded from the website.

Overview of the programme

School Start is a targeted group intervention to boost the language and sound awareness skills of children entering reception class who are delayed in these areas of communication. It also addresses aspects of attention, following instructions and social communication. It aims to help children catch up so that they may be ready to access the learning environment of Year 1. These children are believed to require additional support that is over and above the support that all children receive in the Reception year classroom (universal care).

This provision recognises that children needing targeted support require:

- small group settings to learn new skills with focused adult support
- to learn new skills following the typical sequence of development
- gradual building upon existing skills
- reinforcement and repetition of new skills over a long time frame (one year)
- help to transfer new skills into everyday life.

The programme consists of:

- An initial six-week period so that educational staff may identify children of concern.
- A screening checklist to confirm the identification of those children.
- A structured programme of 30 Language group sessions that teaching assistants will find quick and easy to follow; delivered once a week.
- A structured programme of 30 Sound Awareness group sessions that teaching assistants will find quick and easy to follow; delivered once a week.
- Activities and learning objectives linked into communication at home and in class.
- Monitoring of each child's objectives and re-administration of the checklist in July.

Early Years Foundation Stage profile

School Start is a targeted intervention that is designed to help children achieve the early learning goals described in the Early Years Foundation Stage profile (UK Government, 2014b) by the end of the Foundation Stage. Some of the children in the programme will achieve the early learning goals in this time frame while others will still be working towards the completion of these goals. *School Start* will enable children to develop in the following areas.

- Communication and language development: listening and attention, understanding and speaking.
- Personal, social and emotional development: self-confidence and self-awareness, and making relationships.

Who is involved in delivering the *School Start* programme?

Teaching assistants

School Start is written in such a way that teaching assistants are able to deliver the programme. It is recommended that there are up to six children in a group, led by one teaching assistant. Schools generally prefer to use teaching assistants who are working in the reception class as they are then in the best position to support the transfer of skills learned in the session into the classroom.

Inclusion Coordinator (INCo)

The school's INCo (or Special Educational Needs Coordinator, SENCo) is key to leading the school's commitment to the programme and will allocate time to the teaching assistants to prepare and deliver the programme. The INCo will need to oversee the programme throughout the year to ensure that its operation is smooth: for example, the timetabled slot for the groups and the place where the groups will take place should be kept consistent. The INCo can also take responsibility for evaluating the programme's effectiveness in order to present a case for its continuation in successive years.

Reception class teachers

The reception class teachers will be involved in identifying children they are concerned about at the start of the academic year. They may also help the teaching assistants in completing the Language Sessions Checklist and the Sound Awareness Sessions Checklist. Once the programme is running, the class teacher can increase the programme's effectiveness by helping children to use the new skills they have learned in the classroom (see 'Transferring new skills into the class', page 13).

Speech and language therapists

The programme may be supported in school by the local speech and language therapy team or local authority support services. In this instance, the school may request support to set up the programme, identify the children, deliver the programme and use appropriate signing systems. In some areas this form of support may be given at intervals; for example, the therapist may co-deliver a six-week block of sessions at the start of the programme and then observe a session, giving feedback, later on during the year. There is a sample service agreement, which might be presented by a speech and language therapist or a local authority support service, and a description of the programme in Part 4 (see pages 192–4).

The children

School Start is designed to boost delayed Language and Sound Awareness skills in Reception year children. These children may not have been referred to speech and language therapy or previously identified as having special educational needs. Some may be vulnerable in a range of areas and may also demonstrate difficulties with attention, following instructions and social interaction. *School Start* uses the small group format to promote all aspects of communication to prepare children for the demands of Year 1 (5–6 years).

Children who are delayed or disordered in both speech clarity and language development tend to benefit from both the Language sessions and the Sound Awareness sessions. However, there is often a distinct group of children who have poor speech clarity and sound-processing skills yet have age-appropriate language development; these children will typically only require the Sound Awareness sessions. Where children attend both Language sessions and Sound Awareness sessions, it is beneficial if the groups run on different days.

Children with known speech and language difficulties

Children who are already known to the speech and language therapy service because they have speech, language and communication needs will benefit from *School Start* as a part of their package of specialist intervention. For these children the speech and language therapist may recommend additional forms of support during Reception year. *School Start* is often a good way to settle a child into Reception year before starting further forms of intervention; for some children *School Start* proves to be sufficient intervention to achieve progress.

Occasionally, children known to the speech and language therapy service before Reception year do not meet the criteria for inclusion in the programme using the checklist. These children will have made progress so that they no longer require targeted input and the school may monitor their communication with universal support in the classroom.

Children with additional special educational needs

Children who have known special educational needs, including communication difficulties, may benefit from *School Start* in addition to other forms of specialist provision. Sometimes the extent of a child's difficulties only becomes apparent for the first time in the small group situation of *School Start*. These children may fail to make the expected progress on the programme, relative to the other children. In this instance, the school may like to consider making a referral to their local speech and language therapy department. If the teaching assistants are concerned that the children are not achieving an objective, or are concerned about a particular child's response or behaviour, they should seek advice from the school's INCo. The activity may need to be presented in a different way, to better suit the child's learning style.

Children with difficulties in social communication

Schools sometimes want to include a child with a social communication difficulty (for example, an autism spectrum disorder) in *School Start*. This is because the focus on social skills in the small group could be helpful. However, the potential disruption to the other children needs to be considered. The school will need to decide whether the child has reached a stage of social development at which he may benefit from a group situation: for example, is he able to cooperate in play with one other child? If school staff are in doubt, they may like to ask their speech and language therapist.

Children with English as an additional language

School Start is not recommended for children who have English as an additional language (EAL) or are bilingual, and no other difficulties, because the programme will progress too slowly. However, it can be appropriate when a child has EAL together with other vulnerabilities.

Implementing the programme

Timetable for the year

School Start is designed to be delivered throughout the Reception year as follows.

First half of the autumn term (September–October)

- Children settle into school.
- Children are identified as potentially suitable for the *School Start* Language and/or Sound Awareness group.
- Children are screened using the Language Sessions Checklists and/or the Sound Awareness Sessions Checklist.
- Set-up and training meetings take place between the Inclusion Coordinator (INCo), reception class teachers and teaching assistants.

From the second half of the autumn term until end of the summer term (October–July)

- Language group sessions 1–30 and/or Sound Awareness group sessions 1–30 are delivered weekly in six-week blocks.
- At the end of each six-week block of sessions, the children's progress is recorded for the class teacher and parents or carers.

- At the beginning of each six-week block of sessions, the class teacher is given the learning objectives for this six-week block.

End of the school year (July)

- A Child's Evaluation Record is completed for each child.

- Each child is rescreened using the checklist(s); scores can be compared for a numerical evaluation of individual outcome.

- The checklist scores before and after *School Start* for all the children on the programme can be totalled to demonstrate the effectiveness of the programme.

- The school can plan commitment to delivering *School Start* in the next academic year.

> In some instances a school may want to begin *School Start* at a different point in the school year. This is possible with some replacement of topic vocabulary; for example, replacing the Christmas vocabulary in week 6 with spring or summer vocabulary. However, the programme is written so that the concepts and syntax follow a developmental order and, for this reason, it is best to follow it from week 1 through to week 30. It is not recommended that this resource is 'dipped into' and sessions are applied randomly to children.

First half-term: September–October

Set-up meeting

A meeting between the INCo, reception class teachers and teaching assistants should take place at the start of the academic year. At this meeting, practical arrangements for the programme need to be agreed by the staff involved; this may also involve local support services. There is an agenda for the items to be agreed at this meeting in Part 4 together with a blank *School Start* Timetable to record the arrangements.

It is highly recommended that extra time is allocated during this half-term for making up the picture resources for the first time that the programme is delivered. This ensures that minimal preparation time is needed once the programme is being delivered during the year.

Training meeting

The training meeting is also held in the first six weeks of the academic year. In this meeting, staff prepare themselves for administering the Language Sessions Checklist and Sound Awareness Sessions Checklist and delivering the group sessions; this will involve familiarising themselves with the checklists, Group Session Sheets and other resources. It is also an opportunity to agree how the team will work collaboratively throughout the year. There is an agenda for the items to be discussed at this meeting in Part 4, together with handouts on 'Tips for running the Language Sessions' and 'Tips for running the Sound Awareness Sessions'.

Identification of children: using the checklists

In the first half-term, children are typically settling into their new environment. The educational staff are able to observe the children and form concerns about the communication development of certain children. In addition, the teacher will probably be aware of the children who are already known to have speech and language difficulties from Early Years provisions. These are the children who may then be screened using the checklists for suitability for *School Start*.

There are two checklists:

- the Language Sessions Checklist, which is used to identify children who will benefit from the Language sessions
- the Sound Awareness Sessions Checklist, which is used to identify children who will benefit from the Sound Awareness sessions.

The Reception year class teacher and teaching assistants are best placed to complete the checklists based on their observation of the child in the classroom and as part of their assessment for the Foundation Stage Profile. Some schools prefer to screen the children in a more formal way by setting up a series of play-based activities to challenge the child's understanding and use of the skills in the checklists.

The checklists opposite and overleaf have been designed to require minimal time to complete; it is recommended that no more than 10 minutes is spent on each one. A low total score for 'achieved' items indicates suitability for *School Start*.

Checklist Instructions for Classroom Assistants

Stage 1

- During the first six weeks of Term 1, classroom staff will be getting to know the children.
- Identify those children who are a cause for concern with regard to their speech and language skills. This will be based on your initial impressions, baseline assessments and any background information.

Stage 2

- Complete the checklist for the selected children, as follows.
    - Use the Language Sessions Checklist for children with poor understanding.
    - Use the Sound Awareness Sessions Checklist for children with poor speech clarity and known difficulties with sounds.
- Identify the best person to complete the relevant checklist. For example, it may be the classroom assistant who observes the child and completes the checklist. It would then be good practice for the classroom assistant to discuss the results with the class teacher to

see whether their observations of the child correspond. If there is a difference of opinion, it may be necessary to specifically test an aspect of the child's communication.

- Observe the child at play in class and set up some informal situations to test their skills; for example, give instructions at the sandpit using 'big' and 'little'. Recall how they did and mark it on the checklist.

- Alternatively, you may find it easier to gather together some specific play equipment to test the skills on the checklist more formally. Some suggested toys are as follows.

Language Sessions Checklist Toys:

- coloured, nesting cups
- small coloured bricks or cotton wool balls
- form board with coloured shapes
- collection of familiar items in class – pencils, scissors
- doll or similar that can be made to move – jump, skip, run
- farm animals
- plastic fruit

Sound Awareness Sessions Checklist Toys:

- hoops to put on the floor to step into
- pictures of familiar objects that rhyme; eg cat/hat, dog/frog, fox/box
- pictures of objects with two sounds; eg egg, door, car, bee

- Be aware that some items in the checklists ask if the child 'knows' a concept or can 'follow' an instruction; this is because we are testing understanding. In contrast, some items ask if the child can 'name'; this is because we are testing expressive language.

- The items are arranged in developmental order. For example, a child should be able to detect rhyme before blending spoken sounds. So once a child is unable to show a skill, move on to the next section (ie if a child does not know 'big' and 'little', move on to 'Vocabulary').

- The sum of scores achieved is calculated to decide if the child will benefit from one of the group programmes – either Language or Sound Awareness; some children may need to attend both groups. *School Start* also helps children in the skill areas of attention, following instructions and social interaction. Additional difficulties in these areas can constitute extra cause for including the child in *School Start*.

Language Sessions Checklist

Child's name:	Isobel Smith	Date of birth:	00.00.00
School name:	St Anne's	Class:	???
Completed by:	Mrs Latham, TA	Date of completion:	30 September 20XX
Decision:	Accepted for the group		

Concepts	Rarely (0–40%)	Sometimes (41–80%)	Often (81% +)
A1 Knows big ■ and little ■			X
A2 Names some colours			X
A3 Knows ■ more ☐ no more ☐ before ☐ after ■ first ☐ last		X	
A4 Knows concepts of shapes ☐ ○ △	X		
A5 Knows ■ many ☐ less ■ bigger		X	

Vocabulary	Rarely (0–40%)	Sometimes (41–80%)	Often (81% +)
B1 Can name familiar items in class (eg pencil, scissors) and body parts (eg nose, mouth, legs)			X
B2 Can follow verbal instructions containing actions, eg hop, climb, cut, skip, jump (no use of gesture by the adult)		X	
B3 Can sort objects into two groups according to category (relate to topic work, eg fruit/not fruit; wood/not wood)	X		
B4 Can give five words in a category, eg animals, food	X		
B5 Can give the meaning (function and features) of a topic word recently taught in class, eg What is a mini-beast?	X		
Total of items in column three 'often' = (A score of 4 or less indicates suitability for the group)			3

The following factors may give additional reason for including the child in the Language Group: (circle as appropriate)

Attention	not a concern	⟨a cause for concern⟩
Following instructions	not a concern	⟨a cause for concern⟩
Social interaction	⟨not a concern⟩	a cause for concern

Sound Awareness Sessions Checklist

Child's name:	Isobel Smith	Date of birth:	00.00.00
School name:	St Anne's	Class:	???
Completed by:	Mrs Latham, TA	Date of completion:	30 September 20XX
Decision:	Accepted for the group		

Sound Awareness	Rarely (0–40%)	Sometimes (41–80%)	Often (81% +)
C1 Can walk three steps to show three words in a spoken sentence			✗
C2 Can clap out the syllables in own name		✗	
C3 Can find two pictures of spoken words that rhyme	✗		
C4 Can listen to spoken words and say if they do or do not rhyme	✗		
C5 Can hear two sounds and blend to say the word (eg $e + gg$ = egg)	✗		
Speech	Rarely (0–40%)	Sometimes (41–80%)	Often (81% +)
C6 Speech can be clearly understood by unfamiliar adults	✗		
	Total of items in column three 'often' = (A score of 3 or less indicates suitability for the group)		1

The following factors may give additional reason for including the child in the Sound Awareness Group: (circle as appropriate)

Attention   not a concern   (a cause for concern)

Following instructions   not a concern   (a cause for concern)

Social interaction   (not a concern)   a cause for concern

Planning organisation of the groups

Before the half-term break, it is essential that the class teachers and the teaching assistant who will be delivering the programme agree the practical arrangements for the groups. Successful administration of the programme relies on good planning at this stage that identifies:

- Who will deliver the programme?
- When will the sessions take place?
- Where will the sessions take place?
- Which children will attend which group?

There is a *School Start* timetable template in Part 4 to serve as a written agreement for these arrangements.

Delivering the group sessions: October–July

Each group session offers three activities, which are expected to last up to 30 minutes. Information is given on each Group Session Sheet about learning objectives and materials, including the Resource Templates needed and signs and symbols. The Group Session Sheet also acts as a record sheet for each group session.

The group sessions have been designed so that all three activities may be completed in one session, while maintaining the interest and attention of young children. It is recommended that the first sessions are only 20 minutes long, using all three activities with a short duration, and build up towards a total session time of 30 minutes. In order to maintain the children's concentration, it may be useful to incorporate a physical task between activities, such as asking the children to stand up, hop on one leg, stretch, turn around, etc.

Group Session Sheets

Part 2 contains all of the Group Session Sheets you need to implement *School Start*. These are divided into two areas – Language and Sound Awareness – each containing 30 easy-to-use sheets recommending a variety of different activities. Sample Language Group Session and Sound Awareness Group Session Sheets are provided on pages 13 and 14.

As you will see, the Group Session Sheets can be photocopied and may be used as records of the children's progress during each session. Space is given for you to record information relating to four children on each sheet. If your group contains more than four children, you will need to make *two* photocopies of the Group Session Sheet before the session begins. Each Group Session Sheet lists the Resource Templates needed.

Suggested activities to help children transfer their new skills into class and home are also included on the session sheets; they are denoted by the symbol 🏠.

Sample Group Session Sheets

Language Group Session Sheet   Week 1

Learning objectives
- To work as part of a group taking turns and sharing
- To investigate objects and materials using all of their senses
- To find named item on request (classroom objects)
- To match two pictures that are the same

Date: 23/11/2XXX

Activities	Resources	Names of children and notes on their progress			
		Ann	Oliver	Sarah	Asif
1 A toy is passed around the circle. When the bell rings, whoever is holding the toy says his name.	• Toy such as a teddy, doll or puppet • A bell or other percussion instrument	Whispered	Yes	Yes	Yes
2 Lotto: one board is used and all the pictures are in a bag. Children take turns to take a card and match it to the picture on the board. The adult says that the pictures are 'the **same**' as the child makes a correct match.	• Template 1: Lotto board (1) (two copies, one cut out to make separate cards) • An opaque bag or a box • Scissors	Yes	Yes	Yes, when copying adult's sign	Yes
3 Classroom objects: items are presented and named by the adult. Each child can take turns to feel the items, then the adult asks each child to put a named item in a hoop.	• Seven class objects (eg scissors, pencil, paper, bricks, glue, paint pot, paint brush) • Hoop	Yes	No. Chose item of own interest	Yes Tried to help Oliver	Yes. When adult reduced choice
4 Recap. What did we do **first**? What did we do **next**? What did we do **last**? Show items to give prompts.		Pointed to toy	Said 'pictures'	No response	Looked at objects

Follow-on classroom activity
Table top activity: using two sets of the lotto board cards (Template 1), cut out into individual pictures, the children are asked to find two pictures that are the same.

Sound Awareness Session Sheet

Week 1

Learning objectives
- To listen for a word and respond appropriately
- To identify noises and sounds in the environment
- To join in a familiar nursery rhyme

Date: 23/11/2XXX

Activities	Resources	Names of children and notes on their progress				
		Megan	Oliver	Zafir	Luce	
1 Tell the children that they must each listen for their own name. Each child puts up his hand or stands when he hears it. Once the children become familiar with each other's names, they can take turns to call them out.		No	Yes. Remembered Megan's name	Yes when adult looked	Yes	
2 Sing a familiar nursery rhyme with the children all together, eg 'Humpty Dumpty'. Omit the last rhyming word and see whether the children can supply the missing word.	• A nursery rhyme book with pictures, if available	Yes	Yes	Yes	Yes	
3 Go for a little walk, or stay where you are sitting, and ask the children to listen to the sounds around you for 30 seconds. Then ask the children to tell you what they heard. Draw all of the things you heard on a piece of paper.	• A large piece of paper • A pen or colouring pencil	Yes	Heard the rain	Yes	Heard someone cough	
4 Recap. What did we do **first**? What did we do **next**? What did we do **last**? Show items to give prompts.		Unsure	Unsure	Said 'hands' when prompted with visual reminder	Pointed to book	

Follow-on classroom activity
Sing familiar nursery rhymes. Omit the last word and see whether the children can say the missing word.

Materials

Wherever possible, play the games using real objects and toys found in the classroom. The materials needed for each session are listed on the Group Session Sheet in the column headed 'Resources'. If you do not have some of the objects or toys listed, there is an option to use cut-out cards from the Resource Templates section as an alternative. The same toys are used frequently for the programme, so teaching assistants will find it quicker and easier to collect a box of these toys in readiness for the groups throughout the year to cut down on preparation time.

Resource Templates

There are 70 Resource Templates in total: you will find these in Part 3. Templates 1 to 44 are for the Language sessions and Templates 45 to 70 are for the Sound Awareness sessions. Each template shows the week (or weeks) number in which it is to be used.

The Resource Templates can be photocopied and are to be used in conjunction with the Group Session Sheets. You may want to photocopy some of the templates onto card (eg the lotto boards, picture pairs and syllable cards) and laminate them to ensure that these activities can be used for more than one group.

Some Resource Templates for the Language sessions are suitable for children to take home, and are denoted by the symbol 🏠. These templates are referred to as Home Sheets. For further information, please see the section 'Transferring new skills into the home' on page 14.

Transferring new skills into the class

School Start will be most successful when its learning objectives are extended to the classroom. Class teachers play an important part in facilitating this link. However, because *School Start* is designed to be delivered in small groups that take place outside the classroom, it can be difficult for the class teacher to feel involved with the programme and to ensure that children apply in class their newly acquired skills. There are many ways in which the group sessions may be linked with work in the classroom. Some are described below.

> • The teaching assistant works in both the group and the classroom.

The group sessions are typically delivered by the teaching assistants from the reception class. In this way they can help the children continue to practise their newly acquired skills from the group in the classroom. The teaching assistant also forms a vital communication link with the class teacher, informally updating her of how the children are learning in the group.

> • Handouts for Home and Class and Child Evaluation Records are shared for each six-week block of sessions.
>
> • The teaching assistant and the class teacher arrange a six-weekly meeting to discuss progress with *School Start*.

On a more formal level, the teaching assistant provides the class teacher with the handouts for home and class that contain learning objectives, and Child Evaluation Records for each six-week block of sessions. It is recommended that the teaching assistants and class teachers arrange a time to meet at least once every half-term in order to share information about the programme. This is also an opportunity for the class teacher to suggest topic vocabulary for the Language sessions, which links in with topic work from class. It is suggested that the vocabulary in the programme is used flexibly to reflect the current topic. The equipment and items used in the groups should be made accessible to the children to use during their free play time in the classroom.

- The class teacher takes a group session.
- A group session activity is repeated in the whole class.
- A table top activity is set up that contains an activity from that week's Language session.
- The Makaton® signs used in the group are clearly displayed in class for all staff to see and use.

It is recommended that the class teacher swaps with the teaching assistant on at least one occasion so that she takes the group session, while the teaching assistant takes the rest of the class. This is an invaluable way of helping the class teacher become aware of the provision that the children are receiving. From this understanding often comes a discussion about how to link classroom and group activities: for example, a group activity can be repeated in the whole class. In this way the group children benefit from being the 'experts' in an activity among their peers.

Transferring new skills into the home

Schools will have their own policy regarding informing parents and carers when they include a child in a small group. Some schools choose not to highlight this form of provision as they feel it is just one of many group teaching approaches that they use. If the school wants to inform parents and carers about *School Start*, there is a handout in Part 4 which may be helpful.

When parents or carers are aware that their child is attending *School Start*, it gives the school an opportunity to share with them the child's learning objectives and to keep them informed by means of an ongoing evaluation of the child's progress. It is recommended that parents or carers are also involved in helping their child meet the learning objectives. For instance, the vocabulary and concepts introduced in the group for a particular week can be sent home for reinforcement in real-life situations. In addition, there are handouts for parents and carers in Part 4 'Handouts for home and class'.

Home Sheets

Home Sheets are included in the Resource Templates for use in the Language group sessions. They have been specially designed to be taken home by children so that they may be completed with their parents or carers. This will help to embed the newly learned skill and will provide parents or carers with a practical involvement in their child's progress. It may be helpful to explain to parents or carers, when their child first joins the programme, that they will be given Home Sheets, but that their use is optional. The Home Sheets can be coloured in or cut up as a stimulus and to reinforce the use of topic words.

Sign and symbol systems

It is recommended that *School Start* is used in association with a sign and symbol system such as Makaton, where signs and symbols accompany spoken language (see Walker & Ferris-Taylor, 1998). The school's local speech and language therapy department should be able to give advice on how to obtain training and support before the introduction of sign and symbol systems. Details of training videos and packs for schools are given in the bibliography. There is a list of useful words to sign in Part 4. Words or concepts for which a sign or symbol may be used are highlighted **like this** on the Group Session Sheets.

However, please note that *School Start* can be used effectively even when the school is not familiar with using signs and symbols.

Signing and symbol use with young language-delayed children

Signing is very useful when working with young children who have poor language skills. For example, it can provide a visual indication of general instructions such as 'good listening', 'sit down' and 'stop'. In these instances the signs are a formal way of using gestures. They help to keep consistent the gestures used by different adults and so increase the chance that children will understand what is expected from them.

In *School Start* the children are introduced to new vocabulary and concepts such as 'first', 'middle' and 'last'. It will be easier for the children to learn these new words and concepts if the appropriate sign is used as the speaker says the word.

It is not intended that the teaching assistants sign every word – only the new concepts as they are introduced. Symbol cards are also recommended as another visual method of making abstract language instructions more concrete and lasting.

The sounds that are introduced in the Sound Awareness group sessions can also be made more concrete and visual through the use of a signing system such as *Cued Articulation* (Passey, 1985a, 1985b). Some schools may be familiar with *Jolly Phonics* (Lloyd, 1995a, 1995b); if so, this may be used during the Sound Awareness group sessions. Where a school does not use *Jolly Phonics*, it is recommended that they adopt *Cued Articulation*. This is because it is based on the principles of how sounds are formed in the mouth, and is therefore favoured by speech and language therapists.

Monitoring progress and outcomes: July

A school may evaluate the success of *School Start* in the following two ways.

Child Evaluation Record of progress

Part 4 contains a photocopiable Child Evaluation Record which can be completed as the child finishes each six-week block of sessions. Each learning objective for the six-week block is listed so that skills may be recorded as seen in the group either 'Rarely', 'Sometimes' or 'Often'. It is recommended that the child's booklet is shared with the class teacher and parents or carers after the completion of each six-week block as an ongoing monitoring of progress. Please note that this is a record of the skills displayed within the group and class teachers still have the responsibility to monitor how the child uses these skills in class.

The Child Evaluation Record may form a useful part of the education, health and care plan of a child with special educational needs. For this reason, it is recommended that the Record is shared with the speech and language therapy service, when appropriate.

Post-group checklist

In order to gauge the success of *School Start* as a targeted group intervention in one school, it is recommended that the checklists are re-administered for each child at the end of the programme in July. In this way pre-group and post-group scores for all children may be compared and the percentage of increase calculated. Similarly, it is also useful to compare the items ticked as 'cause for concern' at the bottom of the checklist.

For individual children, the scores achieved on the checklists in July are useful ways of planning any further intervention required in Year 1.

Some children make unexpectedly good progress within the group and no longer appear to need the small group sessions. When this occurs, use the checklist again to confirm your impressions and let the child leave the group.

Using the *School Start* website

The *School Start* website at www.routledge.com/cw/speechmark gives you the opportunity to print out 40 of the Resource Templates in colour. These templates include several group games and activities that can be used in the classroom as part of the Language sessions and the Sound Awareness sessions.

Each Resource Template is listed as it appears in the book by template number and title as well as the week(s) in which it is used (see Part 3, pages 88–9).

The website also includes downloadable copies of the resources in Part 4 which you can print out.

Part 2
Group Session Sheets

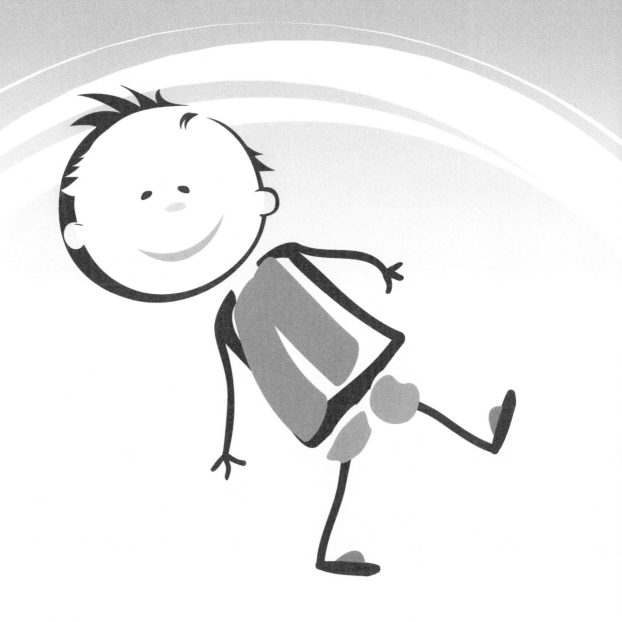

Language Sessions 1–30

Language Group Session Sheet

Week 1

Learning objectives
- To work as part of a group taking turns and sharing
- To investigate objects and materials using all of their senses
- To find named item on request (classroom objects)
- To match two pictures that are the same

Date:		Names of children and notes on their progress				
Activities	**Resources**					
1 A toy is passed around the circle. When the bell rings, whoever is holding the toy says his name.	• Toy such as a teddy, doll or puppet • A bell or other percussion instrument					
2 Lotto: one board is used and all the pictures are in a bag. Children take turns to take a card and match it to the picture on the board. The adult says that the pictures are 'the **same**' as the child makes a correct match.	• Template 1: Lotto board (1) (two copies, one cut out to make separate cards) • An opaque bag or a box • Scissors					
3 Classroom objects: items are presented and named by the adult. Each child can take turns to feel the items, then the adult asks each child to put a named item in a hoop.	• Seven class objects (eg scissors, pencil, paper, bricks, glue, paint pot, paint brush) • Hoop					
4 Recap. What did we do **first**? What did we do **next**? What did we do **last**? Show items to give prompts.						

Follow-on classroom activity
Table top activity: using two sets of the lotto board cards (Template 1), cut out into individual pictures, the children are asked to find two pictures that are the same.

Language Group Session Sheet

Week 2

Learning objectives
- To work as part of a group, taking turns and sharing
- To sustain attentive listening
- To find a named item on request (toy animals or other toys)

Date:

Activities	Resources	Names of children and notes on their progress				
1 Children take turns to roll the ball to each other. Each child says his own name and who he is going to roll it to.	• A ball					
2 Children are given a classroom object to hold. They have to listen for the name of their object and then stand up. If they are good at this, two items can be called and the children have to swap places. Each child can have a turn to be the caller.	• Class objects (eg scissors, pencil, paper, bricks, glue, paint pot, paint brush)					
3 Items are shown and placed in front of the children. Each child takes turns to 'post' the item that the adult names.	• Toy animals or other toys • A box suitable for 'posting' the above items in					
4 Recap. What did we do **first**? What did we do **next**? What did we do **last**? Show items to give prompts.						

Follow-on classroom activity

Role play activity: using classroom objects, set up a pretend shop for children to buy the classroom items. Adults to demonstrate ways to request the items, eg 'Can I have some glue please?'

Language Group Session Sheet

Week 3

Learning objectives
- To work as part of a group taking turns
- To sustain attentive listening
- To follow rules in a group
- To find a named item on request ('big'/'little')

Date:

Activities	Resources	Names of children and notes on their progress				
1 Sing to the tune of 'Frère Jacques': 'Who is sitting? Who is sitting? [Name] is, [Name] is, Come and [activity, eg blow the bubbles], Come and [activity, eg blow the bubbles], Just like this, Just like this.' Then invite a child by name to come and have a turn at the activity of your choice (see resources).	• Marble run, bubbles, bricks or a hat to wear					
2 Each child has to take a card from a bag. If the child picks a **Yes** card, he has a turn at the game; if **No**, he passes on the bag to the next person.	• Template 2: Yes/no cards (cut out to make separate cards) • Scissors • An opaque bag • Game (eg building a tower, lotto game or put a piece in a puzzle)					
3 Show the children **big** and **little** items and symbols on each hoop. Show them that the big items go in one hoop and the little items in the other. Each child chooses an item and places it in the correct hoop. At the end, ask each child to find a 'big …' or 'little …'.	• Template 3: Big and little • Pairs of big and little items • Two hoops • Symbols for 'big' and 'little'					
4 Recap. What did we do **first**? What did we do **next**? What did we do **last**? Show items to give prompts.						

Follow-on classroom activity
Table top activity: using two circles or hoops, stick the big and little symbol onto each one.
Children sort out the big or little objects by placing them in the circle or hoops. Adults comment on other big or little items in the class room.

Language Group Session Sheet

Week 4

Learning objectives
- To sustain attentive listening
- To extend word knowledge (by using 'Yes' / 'No', and the pronoun 'I')

Date:

Activities	Resources	Names of children and notes on their progress				
1 You call out a child's name. The child has to wait for you to say **'Go'** before letting the car roll down the tube. Use the sign for 'Go' if the child has difficulty listening.	• A toy car • A cardboard tube (eg as used for a roll of wrapping paper)					
2 Use **'I'** to refer to self. Take out each food item and name it. Demonstrate the routine (eg 'I like carrots'), then ask each child to tell everyone what they like to eat using 'I'.	• Food items (or Template 4: Food if none are available) • Scissors					
3 **Yes/No** shopping game: name the items as you show them. Ask each child in turn to be the shopkeeper. Ask 'Can I have a ...?' asking for something that is either there or not there. The child has to say 'Yes' or 'No' depending on whether or not they have it.	• Food items (or Template 4: Food if none are available) • Scissors					
4 Recap. What did we do **first**? What did we do **next**? What did we do **last**? Show items to give prompts.						

Follow-on classroom activity
Role play activity: using food items, set up a pretend shop for children to buy the food.
Adults to demonstrate ways to request the food items, eg 'Can I have some cereal please?'

27

Language Group Session Sheet

Week 5

Learning objectives
- To work as part of a group, taking turns and sharing
- To find a named item on request (animals, Christmas vocabulary)
- To extend word knowledge (by using 'a' before an item)

Date:

Activities	Resources	Names of children and notes on their progress				
1 Match the animal sound to the animal. You make the sound (or use recorded animal sounds) and each child finds the animal and names it.	• 'Animal sounds lotto' game or you make the sound and use Template 5: Animals (1)					
2 Christmas items: introduce the items and then ask each child to find a particular item. Then each child chooses an item and names it.	• Christmas objects or Template 6: Christmas					
3 Use 'a' before an item. Ask each child to take out an item from the bag and name it. Tell the children you are going to hide something in the bag. In turns, they have to say what is hiding, using 'a' (eg 'a ball').	• About four interesting objects in an opaque bag, all of them taking the article 'a' (not 'an')					
4 Recap. What did we do **first**? What did we do **next**? What did we do **last**? Show items to give prompts.						

Follow-on classroom activity
Table top activity: colour in and cut out animals from Template 5. Adults to use the animal names frequently while commenting on what the child is doing.

Routledge
Taylor & Francis Group

Language Group Session Sheet

Week 6

Learning objectives

- To work as part of a group taking turns and sharing
- To extend word knowledge (understand and use the concept 'the same')
- To name an item on request (Christmas vocabulary)

Date:

Activities	Resources	Names of children and notes on their progress				
1 Children take turns to build one part of the toy. Then they have to choose who has their turn next by looking at them.	• A Russian doll or a set of building bricks					
2 Using two sets of pictures or objects, place one set in a box and one set in front of the child. Each child chooses an item from the box and matches it with the '**same**' item in front of them. (Make sure the objects are the same size and colour.)	• Pairs of objects or pictures • Box for 'posting' the objects or pictures • Template 7: Which pictures are the same?					
3 Recap on Christmas items. Take an item away and ask each child what is missing.	• Christmas objects or Template 6: Christmas (cut out to make individual pictures) • Scissors					
4 Recap. What did we do **first**? What did we do **next**? What did we do **last**? Show items to give prompts.						

Follow-on classroom activity

Table top activity: colour then cut out the Christmas pictures (Template 6) and stick them on card to make Christmas cards. Adults to name the pictures and repeat these often for children who are not confident naming them.

Language Group Session Sheet

Week 7

Learning objectives
- To be able to arrange items into categories
- To understand the preposition 'on'
- To extend word knowledge (understand and use the word 'and')

Date:

Activities	Resources	Names of children and notes on their progress				
1 Ask the children to sort items into '**furniture**' or '**not furniture**' by placing items in the correct hoop (there should be one for furniture items and one for not furniture items). Then the adult names a furniture item and the child finds it.	• Toy furniture or Template 8: Furniture (cut out into individual pictures) • Other miniature toys (not furniture) or Template 25: Lotto board (2) (cut out into individual pictures) • Two hoops, scissors • Template 9: More furniture 🏠					
2 Place a chair, table and book in front of the children. Show them that we can put items '**on**' these objects (using the sign and symbol). In turns, they all put their hand 'on' something. Then the adult names an item for the child to put 'on' one of the places.	• Chair, table, book, pen, glue, scissors or other items					
3 Shopping game. Explain to the children that they are going to get two items from the shop. They have to say the word '**and**'. Show an example such as 'an apple and a pear'. Tell each child which two items to get and then ask him what he got, encouraging him to say 'and'.	• Food or other items that might come from a shop, or Template 10: More food (cut out into individual pictures) • Scissors					
4 Recap. What did we do **first**? What did we do **next**? What did we do **last**? Show items to give prompts.						

Follow-on classroom activity
Table top activity: using two circles or hoops, stick the 'furniture' and 'not furniture' symbol on each one.
Children sort out the furniture and not furniture objects or pictures by placing them in the circle or hoops.

Language Group Session Sheet

Week 8

Learning objectives
- To find a named item on request (body parts)
- To understand and use the concept 'different'
- To investigate objects and materials using touch
- To extend word knowledge (by asking 'What is it?')

Date:

Activities	Resources	Names of children and notes on their progress					
1 All together in a group, children point to parts of their body that the adult names. Then each child is asked to point to a body part of the doll. Sing 'Head and shoulders, knees and toes'.	• Doll • Template 11: Body parts 🏠						
2 Show a pile of different animals including some that are identical. Tell the children we are looking for animals that are **'different'** to go in the zoo. Use a sign and symbol to show the children two **'different'** animals. Take one animal from the pile and place it in a cage at the zoo. Ask the children in turns to find one that is different to place in the zoo.	• Toy animals (some of which are identical) • Sheet of paper with a drawing of a zoo with lots of cages.						
3 Each child chooses an item to feel and the next child asks **'What is it?'** The child responds, 'It is a ...' Each child has a turn to choose an item.	• Objects in an opaque bag • Blindfold if available or ask the children not to look in the bag						
4 Recap. What did we do **first**? What did we do **next**? What did we do **last**? Show items to give prompts.							

Follow-on classroom activity
Children lie on a large sheet of paper and a friend draws around their body. Encourage the children to name the parts of the body. Adults can comment and name parts of the body that the children are less familiar with.

Language Group Session Sheet

Week 9

Learning objectives
- To understand and use the preposition 'in'
- To extend word knowledge (understand and use the word 'my')
- To find a named item on request (related to kitchenware)

Date:

Activities	Resources	Names of children and notes on their progress					
1 One child chooses an object (from current topic vocabulary) and is asked to put it **'in'** something. You then place the item somewhere and ask the children where it is. Child to respond using 'It is "in" …'.	• Current topic vocabulary items • Places to hide these items in: eg box, bag, shoe						
2 Introduce the word **'my'** with, 'This word tells us things that belong to people, for example 'my jumper'. Each child selects one of their items and says, 'This is my …'	• Collect at least one personal item for each child such as a book, a coat, etc.						
3 Kitchenware (or other topic vocabulary). Name items as you show them to the children. Then ask each child to find something specific. Vary the activity by hiding an object and asking the children, 'What is missing?'	• Kitchenware (eg pan, spoon, scales, tray, whisk, knife, rolling pin, cutter) or Template 12: Kitchenware • Scissors						
4 Recap. What did we do **first**? What did we do **next**? What did we do **last**? Show items to give prompts.							

Follow-on classroom activity
Role play activity: set up an area for pretend cooking. Use play dough as pretend cakes and have the kitchenware items available to play with. Adults to comment on the children's play using the actions such as 'cutting', 'weighing', 'mixing' and naming the kitchenware items, eg 'Oh you're cutting with the knife', 'You're rolling, rolling, with the rolling pin.'

Language Group Session Sheet

Week 10

Learning objectives
- To be able to arrange items into categories
- To understand and use the concept 'first'
- To extend word knowledge (understand and use the word 'mine')

Date:

Activities	Resources	Names of children and notes on their progress				
1 Ask the children to choose an item and sort items into **'toy'** or **'not toy'** by placing them in the correct hoop (there should be one for toys and one for not toys).	• Toys and other items • Template 13: Is it a toy or not?					
2 Children pretend to line up at the bus stop. You ask a child to be **'first'**, then name two other children to line up. You ask, 'Who is first?' The first child puts up his hand. Swap the children around and repeat.						
3 Introduce the word **'mine'** using people's belongings (eg 'The pen is mine'). Put some of the children's belongings into a box. Take out an item and ask, 'Whose is this?' The child who owns the item responds, 'It is mine'.	• Collect at least one personal item for each child, such as a book, coat, etc. • A box					
4 Recap. What did we do **first**? What did we do **next**? What did we do **last**? Show items to give prompts.						

Follow-on classroom activity
For each part of the day use the sign and symbol 'first' to tell the children what they are going to do. Draw a picture of what the first activity will be next to the symbol. This may be a picture of a book for story time for example. At the end of the activities, recap by asking the children 'What did we do first today?' Show the children the symbol and the picture next to it to help them recall the first activity.

Language Group Session Sheet

Week 11

Learning objectives

- To find and name an item on request (clothes)
- To understand the preposition 'under'
- To extend word knowledge (understand and use the word 'your')

Date:

Activities	Resources	Names of children and notes on their progress				
1 Washing **clothes**. Adult shows each item, asking the children what it is and placing it on the washing line. The adult asks the child to find a named item. When all of the washing is collected, each child is asked to name an item.	• Clothes or Template 14: Clothes (cut out into individual pictures) • Scissors • Clothes pegs and string					
2 Children take turns to put their hand **'under'** a chair/table/box. Each child is given an object to place 'under' something and hides the item for the next child. The first child asks, 'Where is the ...?' and the next child responds, 'It is under ....'.	• Random objects • A chair, box and table for hiding the objects under					
3 Using a puppet or toy, explain that it likes to 'land on' people: 'We are going to say where it has landed using the word "**your**" [show the sign and symbol]'. Each child makes it land on someone's clothes or body and says, 'It is on your ...'.	• A puppet or other toy					
4 Recap. What did we do **first**? What did we do **next**? What did we do **last**? Show items to give prompts.						

Follow-on classroom activity

Table top activity: use two sets of the clothes template cut out into individual pictures and laminated. Children take turns to find the matching pairs.
Adults to name the clothes items by commenting on what the children are doing, eg 'You've found a jacket, I wonder if there's another jacket.'
Leave gaps for the children to name the items if they can, eg 'Oh it's a ....'

Week 12

Language Group Session Sheet

Learning objectives
- To extend word knowledge (understand and use the word 'you')   • To extend word knowledge (understand and use regular plural forms such as 'book'/'books')
- To understand and use the concept 'last'

Date:

Activities	Resources	Names of children and notes on their progress				
1 Picnic game: Mum is giving everyone some food. She chooses an item to give to each child, saying 'The ... is for **you**'. Each child takes a turn to be Mum.	• Pretend food and plates					
2 Three children pretend to line up at the ice-cream van. Ask the person who is '**last**' to put up his hand. Then arrange the toy animals as if they are lining up for a drink. (Line up animals facing left from the child's view as in reading words from left to right.) Ask the children to find which animal is 'last'.	• Toy animals					
3 Introduce that when we say a word it is usually one item and if we add an 's' to the end it tells us there are many items. Show a pile of items and say the singular word – taking one item. Then say the plural version and take lots of them. Ask each child to listen carefully and take either one or many.	• Toy animals or pieces of fruit (where the plural version takes an 's'), eg bananas, cars, trains, pears, boats, apples					
4 Recap. What did we do **first**? What did we do **next**? What did we do **last**? Show items to give prompts.						

Follow-on classroom activity
When the children are lining up, explain that the last person has to look after the line. Use the sign and symbol for 'last' and ask the children 'Who is last in line?'

Language Group Session Sheet

Week 13

Learning objectives
- To find a named item on request (parts of a house)
- To understand the concepts 'big', 'middle' and 'little' in relation to size
- To extend word knowledge (understand and use the words 'he' and 'she')

Date:

Activities	Resources	Names of children and notes on their progress				
1 Ask each child to find a particular part of the house. Then invite each child to point to a part and tell the group what it is called. This can be substituted with any other topic work being covered.	• Doll's house or picture of a house • Template 15: Parts of a house					
2 Teddy Bears' Picnic: introduce the different-sized bears – **big**, **little** and **middle**-sized. Ask each child to give some food to either the big, little or middle-sized bear.	• Food items or Template 4: Food and Template 10: More food • Scissors • Three different-sized bears or Template 16: Three sized bears					
3 Introduce the idea that we can use the word '**he**' to talk about a boy and '**she**' to talk about a girl. Using pictures of boys and girls doing actions, ask each child to sort the pictures into 'he' or 'she'. The pictures can be stuck to skittles and, when they knock the skittle over, the child has to pick it up and describe the picture using 'he' or 'she'.	• Template 17: Actions (1) (cut out into cards) • Scissors • Skittles or fishing game					
4 Recap. What did we do **first**? What did we do **next**? What did we do **last**? Show items to give prompts.						

Follow-on classroom activity
Use the story of 'Goldilocks and the Three Bears'. Emphasise the concepts of big, little and middle-sized.

Language Group Session Sheet

Week 14

Learning objectives
- To find and name an item on request (light sources)
- To understand and use the concept 'bigger'
- To extend word knowledge (understand and use regular plurals)

Date:

Activities	Resources	Names of children and notes on their progress		
1 Introduce **'light'** and talk about how we get light from many things. Using pictures or items, name each light source. Then give one to each child to hold. As you call out an item the child has to hold it up. Then play a game in which the child has to find an item and name it, eg taking items from a bag or attaching a paper clip to the picture and using a magnet to fish for it.	- Examples of light sources or Template 18: Light sources (cut out into individual pictures) - Scissors - Bag or fishing game - Template 18: Light sources			
2 Using three pictures of different-sized bears, each child is given two bears to compare. Ask the child to find the bear that is **'bigger'**. Then select two bears and point to the bigger one while asking the child 'Tell me about this one, it is …'	- Three different-sized bears or Template 16: Three sized bears - Scissors			
3 Using the singular or plural template, the adult names an item and the child puts a counter on that picture. When the board is complete, each child takes off a counter and names the picture.	- Counters - Template 19: Singular/plural lotto			
4 Recap. What did we do **first**? What did we do **next**? What did we do **last**? Show items to give prompts.				

Follow-on classroom activity
Table top activity: draw a picture of a fish on a piece of paper. The task is for the children to draw one that is bigger. You could substitute the fish for an item linked to the class topic.

Language Group Session Sheet

Week 15

Learning objectives
- To arrange items into categories according to the materials that they are made from
- To understand the preposition 'behind'
- To extend word knowledge (understand and use the words 'his' and 'her')

Date:		Names of children and notes on their progress					
Activities	**Resources**						
1 Introduce the fact that some things are made of **wood**. (Show the symbol and use the sign.) Demonstrate by placing an item made of wood into one hoop and another item **not wood** in the other. Each child has a turn to choose an item and place it in the correct hoop.	• Objects, some of which are made out of wood and some which are not (eg wooden train, wooden brick, wooden ruler, cup, paint pot, pen) • Two hoops						
2 Using objects to stand behind, demonstrate '**behind**', showing the symbols and using the sign. Each child has a turn to stand behind an item that you name.	• Chair, easel, desk or other objects to stand behind						
3 Using pictures of a boy and a girl, explain that they need clothes to wear. We say 'his clothes' when items belong to a boy and 'her clothes' when items belong to a girl. Each child chooses an item of clothing and decides whether it is 'his clothes' or 'her clothes'.	• Template 20: Boy and girl • Items of clothes or Template 14: Clothes (cut out into individual pictures) • Scissors • Children to take templates home to put clothes on a boy and a girl						
4 Recap. What did we do **first**? What did we do **next**? What did we do **last**? Show items to give prompts.							

Follow-on classroom activity
Table top activity: using two circles or hoops, stick the 'wood' and 'not wood' symbol on each one.
Children sort out the wood and not wood objects or pictures by placing them in the circle or hoops.

Language Group Session Sheet

Week 16

Learning objectives
- To arrange items into categories according to the materials that they are made from
- To understand and use the concepts 'quick' and 'slow'
- To extend word knowledge (by using 'and' to link two verbs together)

Date:		Names of children and notes on their progress				
Activities	**Resources**					
1 Introduce the fact that some things are made of metal. (Show the symbol and use the sign.) Demonstrate by placing an item made of **metal** in one hoop and another made of **not metal** item in the other. Each child has a turn to choose an item and place it in the correct hoop.	• Two hoops • Objects, some of which are made out of metal					
2 Demonstrate that a car can be '**quick**' or '**slow**' when it moves. Each child has to listen for the adult to say how it will move, then the child makes it move appropriately. Each child can tell the next child how to move it.	• A toy car					
3 Each child chooses **two** action pictures and tells everyone what they are, using the verbs and the word '**and**', eg 'walking and drinking'.	• Template 21: Actions (2); see also Template 17: Actions (1) (cut out into cards) • Scissors					
4 Recap. What did we do **first**? What did we do **next**? What did we do **last**? Show items to give prompts.						

Follow-on classroom activity
During a PE lesson, give the children instructions to move in a 'quick' or 'slow' way. Hold up the symbols as you say them.

Language Group Session Sheet

Week 17

Learning objectives

- To arrange items into the categories 'fruit' and 'not fruit'
- To understand and use the preposition 'in front of'
- To ask a question using 'Who?'

Date:		Names of children and notes on their progress				
Activities	**Resources**					
1 Using different foods, explain that you want the children to sort out those that are '**fruit**' and '**not fruit**'. Each child chooses an item and tells you whether it is 'fruit' or 'not fruit'.	• Food including fruit and not fruit, or Template 22: Fruit and Template 24: Vegetables (cut out into individual pictures if objects are not available)					
2 Using the sign and symbol, show the children the concept '**in front**'. They all take turns to sit on a pretend train. The adult tells them who to sit in front of, and then asks them to say where they are sitting using 'in front of'.	• Chairs, arranged to make a pretend train					
3 Using action pictures, name each action. Ask each child, '**Who** is …ing?' Each child should identify the correct picture. Then ask each child to ask the next person a question, '**Who** is …ing?'	• Template 17: Actions (1) and/or Template 21: Actions (2) (cut out to make cards)					
4 Recap. What did we do **first**? What did we do **next**? What did we do **last**? Show items to give prompts.						

Follow-on classroom activity

When the children are lining up, ask them to change places by asking them to stand 'in front of …'. Ask some children to tell you who is in front of them.

Language Group Session Sheet

Week 18

Learning objectives

- To arrange items into the categories 'plastic' and 'not plastic'
- To ask a question using 'Where?'
- To extend word knowledge (using 'no' with a noun)

Date:

Activities	Resources	Names of children and notes on their progress			
1 Use a variety of items to explain that you want the children to sort out those that are 'plastic' and 'not plastic'. Show the children which hoop is for 'plastic' and which is for 'not plastic'. Each child chooses an item and tells you whether it is 'plastic' or 'not plastic', putting it into the correct hoop.	• Plastic and non-plastic items • Two hoops				
2 Make a picture of a face or body, asking the children to tell you what parts you need to add. Then make a face or body with something missing. Each child is to say 'he has …'.	• Template 23: Missing parts (cut out to make separate cards) • Scissors				
3 Tell the children that we ask '**Where**?' when we are trying to find something. Each child has a turn to look away while the other children hide a teddy. The child then chooses someone to ask, 'Where is Teddy?' The chosen child says where Teddy is.	• Small teddy bear				
4 Recap. What did we do **first**? What did we do **next**? What did we do **last**? Show items to give prompts.					

Follow-on classroom activity

Hide a familiar toy or object in the classroom, asking the children 'Where is the …?' The children could take turns to hide the item while everyone else closes their eyes. Then they ask 'Where is the …?' This is a fun game that could be played during a carpet time session.

Language Group Session Sheet

Week 19

Learning objectives
- To arrange items into categories ('vegetables' and 'not vegetables')
- To understand the use of the preposition 'above'
- To extend word knowledge (asking 'What is it?')

Date:

Activities	Resources	Names of children and notes on their progress				
1 Using different foods, explain that you want the children to sort out those that are '**vegetables**' and '**not vegetables**'. Each child chooses an item and tells you whether it is a vegetable or not, placing it in the correct hoop.	• Food items (vegetables and other foods) • Two hoops • Template 24: Vegetables					
2 Using the sign and symbol, show the children '**above**' by placing an item in a box above another item in a box. Each child has a turn to place the items above another one. Then, using a board or piece of paper, draw a line and ask the children to draw something above the line.	• Three boxes stacked on top of each other • Items to put in the boxes • Board or paper and pen					
3 Using a lotto board, each child takes a picture and the next child asks them '**What** is it?' The child tells them what it is and then matches it to the picture on the lotto board.	• Lotto board or Template 25: Lotto board (2) (two copies, one cut out to make separate cards) • Scissors					
4 Recap. What did we do **first**? What did we do **next**? What did we do **last**? Show items to give prompts.						

Follow-on classroom activity
Table top activity: colour in and then cut out the vegetables from Template 24.

Language Group Session Sheet

Week 20

Learning objectives
- To find a named item on request (tools)
- To understand the concepts 'top' and 'bottom'
- To extend word knowledge and use (asking 'Is it ...?')

Date:

Activities	Resources	Names of children and notes on their progress				
1 Each child chooses a tool and shows the others how to use it. The child or adult names the item. Then each child is asked to find a tool that the adult names.	• Toy tools if available or Template 26: Tools, cut out to make separate cards • Scissors					
2 Using a toy man and a ladder, introduce and show the **'top'** and the **'bottom'**. Each child has to listen and put the man in the right place on the ladder.	• Toy man and toy ladder					
3 Show the children pictures of the actions and name the actions. All do the actions together. Then turn the cards over and hide the pictures. Each child chooses a picture and does the action. The other children take turns to ask 'Is it ...?'	• Template 27: Actions (3), cut out to make separate cards (you could also use Templates 17 and 21) • Scissors					
4 Recap. What did we do **first**? What did we do **next**? What did we do **last**? Show items to give prompts.						

Follow-on classroom activity
Place the action cards on a table for the children to play charades. They can take a card and do the action. Their friend guesses what the picture is.

Language Group Session Sheet

Week 21

Learning objectives
- To find two named items on request (toy baby animals)
- To understand the concepts 'full' and 'empty'
- To extend word knowledge of the pronouns 'him' and 'her'

Date:

Activities	Resources	Names of children and notes on their progress				
1 Ask each child to find the animal that you name and put it in the farm or field. When putting the toys away, ask each child to find two of them (eg 'Pass me the lamb and the calf').	• Toy baby animals and a toy field or farm • Template 28: Baby animals					
2 Using sand or water and a container, demonstrate making the containers '**full**' and '**empty**'. Then ask each child to describe one of the containers.	• Sand or water • Two containers – one full, one empty • Cloth and/or dustpan to deal with spillages					
3 Using food items, pretend to have a picnic. If possible, get at least one boy and one girl from the group involved in the picnic. If you have a same-gender group, use a picture of a boy and a girl. Explain to the group that when something is for a boy we can say 'It is for **him**' and we say 'It is for **her**' when it is for a girl. Each child chooses an item of food and gives it to the boy or girl saying 'It is for him/her'.	• Food items (or Templates 4 and 10 cut out into individual pictures) • Scissors					
4 Recap. What did we do **first**? What did we do **next**? What did we do **last**? Show items to give prompts.						

Follow-on classroom activity
Bury the toy baby animals in the sand so the children can dig them out. Adults to model the names of the animals and encourage the children to name them if they can, eg 'Oh it's a ...'. Another version could be to match the animals with their babies.

Language Group Session Sheet

Week 22

Learning objectives
- To investigate objects and materials using touch (shapes)
- To find and name an item on request (in relation to shapes)
- To understand the concepts 'push' and 'pull'
- To extend word knowledge of the pronoun 'yours'

Date:

Activities	Resources	Names of children and notes on their progress				
1 Show the children the **shapes** and name them. Ask each child to choose one and put it in the bag. Then name a shape and ask each child to feel and find it. When all of the shapes have been taken out, take one away and ask each child what is missing.	• Opaque bag filled with common 2D geometric shapes, or Template 29: Shapes (cut out into eight cards) • Scissors					
2 Explain that you are going to sort out the items that you **push** and **pull** into two hoops. Using classroom items that you 'push' or 'pull', each child chooses an item and places it in the correct hoop.	• Classroom items that you push or pull (eg hole punch, stapler, button on toy, button and thread, cap on pen) • Two hoops					
3 Each child has a mini lotto board of four pictures (cut templates into two lengthways). Put all the individual pictures in a bag. Each child takes a picture and says which child it belongs to and then says 'It is **yours**'.	• Lotto boards and cards or two copies of one of the lotto board templates (eg Template 1, 25, 30) • Scissors • An opaque bag					
4 Recap. What did we do **first**? What did we do **next**? What did we do **last**? Show items to give prompts.						

Follow-on classroom activity
Table top activity: the children make a picture out of the shapes or draw around them to make a picture. Adult names the shapes as the child uses them and asks the child to name some of the shapes.

Language Group Session Sheet

Week 23

Learning objectives
- To sustain attentive listening
- To find a named item on request (animals)
- To understand the concept 'below'
- To extend word knowledge of 'an' before a noun beginning with a vowel

Date:

Activities	Resources	Names of children and notes on their progress				
1 Show pictures of animals and give each child one to hold. When a child hears their animal name, he has to stand up. Then place all of the animal pictures in front of the children and ask each child to find one that you name.	• Template 31: Animals (2) (cut out to make eight cards) • Scissors					
2 Show the children **'below'** by placing an item in a box below another of the items in a box. Each child has a turn to place an item below another one. Then draw a line on a board or piece of paper and ask the children to draw a shape below the line.	• Three boxes • Random items that will fit in the boxes • Board or paper					
3 What is missing? Using objects, explain that we use 'an' before a word that begins with a vowel, as do the names of these items. Then hide an item and ask each child what is missing, encouraging them to say 'an ....'	• Objects with names that begin with a vowel sound (eg orange, egg, elephant, apple)					
4 Recap. What did we do **first**? What did we do **next**? What did we do **last**? Show items to give prompts.						

Follow-on classroom activity
Table top activity: place the objects that begin with a vowel in a bag. Children feel the item and guess what it is. Adults model using 'an' before the word, eg 'It's an egg'.

Language Group Session Sheet

Week 24

Learning objectives
- To name items (baby animals)
- To arrange items into categories of the materials they are made from
- To extend word knowledge (use 'It is …' when describing something)

Date:

Activities	Resources	Names of children and notes on their progress				
1 Ask the children to match the baby animal with the parent. (Use toy items rather than cards where possible.) Encourage the children to name the baby animals. If using pictures, name the parent and ask the children to find its baby.	• Toy animals and baby animals • Template 28: Baby animals (may be cut out to make eight cards) • Scissors					
2 Explain that you are going to put items that are made of **paper** into one hoop and items that are **not paper** into the other hoop. Ask each child to place each item into the correct hoop.	• Items made of paper and not paper • Two hoops					
3 Using a range of different coloured items, show the children all of the items, then place them in a bag. Each child looks in the bag and describes an item by its colour (eg 'It is …'). Then the other children try to guess what the item is.	• Items of different colours (eg red car, blue pencil, yellow ball, green cup) • An opaque bag					
4 Recap. What did we do **first**? What did we do **next**? What did we do **last**? Show items to give prompts.						

Follow-on classroom activity
Create a display of things made out of paper. Ask the children to bring in items from home that are made out of paper.

Language Group Session Sheet

Week 25

Learning objectives
- To find and name an item on request (things at the farm)
- To identify items within a given category
- To perform two actions in order ('first …', 'then …')

Date:

Activities	Resources	Names of children and notes on their progress				
1 Introduce the topic 'the farm'. Talk about what you might see at the farm. Ask each child to choose a picture and say what it is and what it is for. Then ask each child to find a picture that you name. Take one picture away: can the children tell you what is missing?	• Template 32: The farm (copied and cut out to make eight cards) • Scissors					
2 Tell the children they are going to do some actions for you but they must do them in the correct order. First, demonstrate the actions; then, tell each child to 'Do … **first, then** …'	• Ideas for actions: point to …, jump, stand, knock, wave, kneel, yawn, dance, hop					
3 Place the picture cards face-down. Ask the children to take a card. You name a category, eg 'fruit', and if a child has a card from that category, he calls out 'Me!' or 'I do!'	• Template 33: Category cards (1) (cut out to make eight separate cards) • Scissors					
4 Recap. What did we do **first**? What did we do **next**? What did we do **last**? Show items to give prompts.						

Follow-on classroom activity:
During carpet time as a warm-up activity, ask the children to do two actions in the correct order, eg 'Do … first, then …' To make this harder, ask the children to wait until you say 'Go'. To make it easier, show the children the actions as you say them.

Language Group Session Sheet

Week 26

Learning objectives

- To find and name parts of a tree
- To extend word knowledge (understand the meaning of 'happy' and 'sad')
- To remember two items after a short time delay

Date:		Names of children and notes on their progress					
Activities	**Resources**						
1 Go outside if possible and look at the parts of a tree. Point to and label each part. Go back inside and look at the pictures. Ask each child to find the picture of the part you name. Turn the pictures face-down and ask each child to choose a picture and name the part.	• Template 34: Parts of a tree • Scissors	✗					
2 Show the children the pictures of **'happy'** and **'sad'**, demonstrating the facial expressions that match. Leave one happy and one sad card showing but turn the others face-down. Each child takes a card without showing the others and makes the facial expression shown on it for the next child. That child then points to the correct picture.	• Template 35: Happy/sad cards (cut out to make eight cards) • Scissors						
3 Set up a pretend toy shop a short walk from where the group is seated. Choose a child to be the shopkeeper. Ask each child to go and buy two items. They must ask the shopkeeper for the items and not just take them. If this is easy, try three items.	• A 'shop' area • Toys (at least four items) • A bag to use as a shopping bag						
4 Recap. What did we do **first**? What did we do **next**? What did we do **last**? Show items to give prompts.							

Follow-on classroom activity

Set up a pretend toy shop in the role play area. Adults could request two or three items to buy from the shop and see whether the child can go to the shop and remember all of the items.

Language Group Session Sheet

Week 27

Learning objectives
- To find and name parts of a plant
- To extend word knowledge (understand the meaning of 'happy' and 'sad')
- To name an item in a given category when given a description

Date:		Names of children and notes on their progress					
Activities	**Resources**						
1 Using a living **plant**, talk about all of its different parts. Each child has a turn to point to the part that you name. Then ask each child to choose a part to point to and name it.	• A living plant • Template 36: Parts of a plant						
2 Each child is told about a situation. They have to point to the correct feeling for that situation, pointing to the '**happy**' or '**sad**' picture. (Situations: falling over, getting a present, going swimming, playing a game, feeling sick, breaking a toy, spilling a drink.)	• Template 35: Happy/sad cards (cut out to make eight cards) • Scissors						
3 Divide the children into two teams. Describe the first object from the description clues provided and choose a child in one team to guess what it is. If the child gets it right, he earns a point. Then describe the next item for someone in the other team.	• Template 37: Description clues						
4 Recap. What did we do **first**? What did we do **next**? What did we do **last**? Show items to give prompts.							

Follow-on classroom activity
Bring a living plant into the classroom and leave the pictures from Template 36 next to it. Invite the children to choose a picture and find the same part on the plant.

Week 28

Language Group Session Sheet

Learning objectives
- To find and name an item on request (at the seaside)
- To identify items within a given category
- To extend word knowledge (ask 'Who?')

Date:

Activities	Resources	Names of children and notes on their progress				
1 Introduce the topic 'the seaside' and talk about what you might see there. Using the pictures, name them and ask each child to find one that you say. Then place the pictures in a pile next to a hoop. Each child throws a beanbag into the hoop and names the picture on top of the pile.	• Template 38: Seaside (copied and cut out to make eight cards) • Scissors • Beanbag • Hoop					
2 Ask a child to select a category card. Then each child in turn names one item in that category. When no more items can be thought of, ask a child to choose another category card.	• Template 39: Category cards (2) (copied and cut out to make eight cards) • Scissors					
3 Show the children that some pictures on the cards are the same. Deal out the cards to all the children, making sure they do not have two the same. Each child has to ask 'Who has the …?' to find the same picture. The second child hands over his matching picture and then has his turn.	• Template 40: Picture pairs (1) and Template 41: Picture pairs (2) (cut out into individual pictures) • Scissors					
4 Recap. What did we do **first**? What did we do **next**? What did we do **last**? Show items to give prompts.						

Follow-on classroom activity
Table top activity: using the category cards, the children can draw or paint lots of things belonging to that category on a sheet of paper.

Language Group Session Sheet

Week 29

Learning objectives

- To find and name an item on request (clothes for a hot day)
- To understand the concept 'many'
- To use the structure 'It is not' in sentences

Date:

Activities	Resources	Names of children and notes on their progress
1 Introduce the idea that **clothes** can keep us warm or cool. Look at what sort of day it is today and what clothes the children came to school in. Using the picture cards or real clothes, ask the children to select the clothes that someone might wear on a hot day.	• Clothes from lost property or Template 42: Clothes for a hot day and Template 43: Clothes for a cold day (cut out into individual pictures) • Scissors	
2 Introduce the concept '**many**' and show the children a container with many items in it and one with only a few. Empty the two containers and place different numbers of items into each one. Ask each child which one contains 'many'.	• Two containers • Small items, eg counters, to fit in the containers	
3 Show the children five pictures and name each one. Then turn the pictures over and ask each child to choose a picture card without showing the others. The other children have to guess what it is. If they are not correct, the child has to say 'It is **not** …'.	• Five random pictures such as from Template 1: Lotto board (1) (cut out into individual pictures)	
4 Recap. What did we do **first**? What did we do **next**? What did we do **last**? Show items to give prompts.		

Follow-on classroom activity

Place different amounts of counters or cubes in a container. One container has a few and the other has many. Use the symbol 'many' with the written question 'Which one has many?' Adults to prompt the children to find and name the one with 'many'. The children can empty the containers and then make one contain 'many'.

Language Group Session Sheet

Week 30

Learning objectives
- To understand vocabulary related to body parts
- To understand and use the terms 'here' and 'there'
- To understand and use the word 'or' in a sentence

Date:

Names of children and notes on their progress					

Activities	Resources
1 Introduce the concept of body parts. With the group, name and point to each **body** part. Then each child has a turn to point to a part of their own body. (Extend this by asking the children to point to two body parts in the correct order, or ask the children to tell each other which parts to point to.)	• Template 44: Parts of your body
2 Select items that belong to the area where you are sitting and items from a place still visible but further away. Using the sign and symbol, introduce the words '**here**' and '**there**'. Each child chooses an item and tells you whether it belongs here or there.	• Items from the area you are in and nearby
3 Introduce the word 'or', which tells us we can choose. Play a game giving each child an instruction to choose a colour (eg red or yellow). When each child has had his turn, he can ask the next child to choose, using 'or' as previously.	• Game such as building bricks or throwing a coloured ball into a hoop
4 Recap. What did we do **first**? What did we do **next**? What did we do **last**? Show items to give prompts.	

Follow-on classroom activity
Sing the song 'Head and shoulders, knees and toes'.

Sound Awareness
Sessions 1–30

Sound Awareness Session Sheet

Week 1

Learning objectives
- To listen for a word and respond appropriately
- To identify noises and sounds in the environment
- To join in with a familiar nursery rhyme

Date:

Activities	Resources	Names of children and notes on their progress				
1 Tell the children that they must each listen for their own name. Each child puts up his hand or stands when he hears it. Once the children become familiar with each other's names, they can take turns to call them out.						
2 Sing a familiar nursery rhyme with the children all together, eg 'Humpty Dumpty'. Omit the last rhyming word and see whether the children can supply the missing word.	• A nursery rhyme book with pictures, if available					
3 Go for a little walk, or stay where you are sitting, and ask the children to listen to the sounds around you for 30 seconds. Then ask the children to tell you what they heard. Draw all of the things you heard on a piece of paper.	• A large piece of paper • A pen or colouring pencil					
4 Recap. What did we do **first**? What did we do **next**? What did we do **last**? Show items to give prompts.						

Follow-on classroom activity
Sing familiar nursery rhymes. Omit the last word and see whether the children can say the missing word.

Week 2

Sound Awareness Session Sheet

Learning objectives
- To listen for a word and respond appropriately
- To join in with a familiar nursery rhyme
- To identify which instrument is played from a choice of two

Date:		Names of children and notes on their progress				
Activities	**Resources**					
1 The children stand in a row and when they hear their own name they have to jump one space forwards. If you have a Twister® mat, they can jump on the spots, or in the hoops.	• Twister® mat or hoops, if available					
2 Pass the two instruments around the circle and let the children play each of them. Then ask each child in turn to close their eyes or hide the instruments behind a board and make a sound using one of them. Each child has to listen and identify the instrument.	• Two musical instruments (eg tambourine, jingle bells, clappers, recorder) • A board to hide them behind					
3 Sing a familiar nursery rhyme with the children all together (eg 'Twinkle, twinkle, little star'). Omit the last rhyming word and see whether the children can supply it.	• A nursery rhyme book with pictures, if available					
4 Recap. What did we do **first**? What did we do **next**? What did we do **last**? Show items to give prompts.						

Follow-on classroom activity
During story time, ask the children to listen for a particular word. When they hear it, they clap their hands.

Sound Awareness Session Sheet

Week 3

Learning objectives
- To listen for a word and respond appropriately
- To identify which musical instrument is played from a choice of two

Date:

Activities	Resources	Names of children and notes on their progress			
1 Each child is given an item to hold. Check that each child knows the name of the item. Call out the name of one item. When the child hears the name of his item, he holds it up. If the children are good at this, two items can be called out and the children holding the items have to swap places.	• Classroom objects for each child to hold, eg: paper, pencil, eraser, ruler, paper clip, small toys				
2 Items are placed in front of the children. Each child in turn has to listen for the name of the item and 'post' it in the box or hoop.	• Objects such as paper, pencil, eraser, ruler, paper clip, small toys • Box or a hoop through which the objects can be 'posted'				
3 Each child closes his eyes or turns around while you play one of the musical instruments. They have to listen and identify the instrument from a choice of two.	• Two musical instruments				
4 Recap. What did we do **first**? What did we do **next**? What did we do **last**? Show items to give prompts.					

Follow-on classroom activity
During a PE lesson, tell the children to move around and when they hear the bell, they have to 'freeze'.

Sound Awareness Session Sheet

Week 4

Learning objectives
- To listen for a word and respond appropriately
- To join in with a familiar nursery rhyme
- To understand the concept 'first'

Date:

Activities	Resources	Names of children and notes on their progress			
1 Each child in turn listens and waits for you to say 'Go' and then rolls the ball down the tube.	• Cardboard tube (eg from a roll of wrapping paper) • A small ball that fits easily inside the tube				
2 Sing a familiar nursery rhyme with the children (eg 'Jack and Jill'). Replace the rhyming word and see whether the child can tell you what it should be (eg 'Jack and Jill went up the wall').					
3 Introduce the concept **'first'** using the sign and symbol. Explain to the children that they are going to take turns to line up at the bus stop. They have to listen to find out who will be first. Call out the first name, then two others. Ask the first child to put up his hand. Then mix up the children and repeat, asking, 'Now who is "first"?'	• Pretend bus stop				
4 Recap. What did we do **first**? What did we do **next**? What did we do **last**? Show items to give prompts.					

Follow-on classroom activity:
When the children are lining up, use the sign and symbol for 'first' and ask the children 'Who is first in line?'

Sound Awareness Session Sheet

Week 5

Learning objectives

- To listen for a sound and respond appropriately
- To be aware of words that rhyme
- To understand the concept 'first'

Date:

Activities	Resources	Names of children and notes on their progress				
1 While each child listens for the sound 's', you make different sounds. When he hears an 's', he posts a counter in the box. Make the sound with the *Cued Articulation* sign, and then without it.	• Counters • Box suitable for posting counters in • *Cued Articulation* sign for 's'					
2 Tell the children that together you are going to think of some words that rhyme, such as 'incy', 'wincy', 'pincy'. Ask the children if they can think of any words that rhyme. Use the children's names to give examples, and offer a nonsense word that rhymes and one that does not. Ask each child to tell you which word rhymes with their name and to give their own words that rhyme.						
3 Recap on last week's lining-up activity. This time, the children are to line up at the sweet shop. Line them up and ask the child who is **first** to put up his hand. Then line up three different toy animals going for a drink of water. Ask each child which animal is **first**.	• Three different toy animals • Blue paper to represent water • Items for a pretend sweet shop					
4 Recap. What did we do **first**? What did we do **next**? What did we do **last**? Show items to give prompts.						

Follow-on classroom activity

During carpet time, explain that you are going to think of some silly rhymes with the children's names. Give some examples, eg Mo, Vo; Ella, Mella. When asking the children to get up, use a rhyme with their name.

Sound Awareness Session Sheet

Week 6

Learning objectives
- To be able to listen for a sound and respond appropriately
- To be aware of words that rhyme
- To understand the concept 'last'

Date:

Activities	Resources	Names of children and notes on their progress					
1 Each child has to listen for a 'p' sound. The adult demonstrates by making different sounds, and when a 'p' sound is made, the children take it in turns to add a brick to the tower.	• Bricks that can be built into a tower • *Cued Articulation* sign for 'p' – use initially with sound then without						
2 Introduce some characters and give each one a silly name. Ask the children to think of a word that rhymes with the character's name (eg 'fuzzy', 'buzzy', 'muzzy'). If the children are unable to give an example, offer some words that rhyme and some that do not. Can they tell you whether the two words rhyme or not?	• Pictures of monsters or Lego® robots						
3 Introduce the concept **'last'** using the sign and symbol. Explain that three children are going to line up to post letters. Call out three of the children's names and ask them to line up. Then ask the child who is last to put up his hand. Mix up the children and ask again who is last.	• Letter box • Pretend letters for posting						
4 Recap. What did we do **first**? What did we do **next**? What did we do **last**? Show items to give prompts.							

Follow-on classroom activity
During carpet time, ask the children to listen to the two words you say. They have to put up their hand if they think it rhymes. Use your own name and some words that rhyme and some that do not, eg Davis, Pavis and Davis, Leeb.

Sound Awareness Session Sheet

Week 7

Learning objectives
- To listen for a sound from a choice of two and respond appropriately
- To identify which words rhyme
- To understand the concept 'last'

Date:	Resources	Names of children and notes on their progress				
Activities	**Resources**					
1 Each child has to listen for a 'p' or an 's' sound. When he identifies one of these sounds, he has to roll the car down the correct tube.	• Two cardboard tubes • The letters 'p' and 's', for sticking on each tube					
2 Explain that you are going to say two words. The child has to tell you whether they rhyme or sound alike, eg: 'me' and 'bee', 'chair' and 'duck'. Ask the child to point to the yes/no or happy/sad face.	• Template 45: Yes/no or happy/sad faces					
3 Introduce the concept **'last'** using the symbol and sign. Choose a child to be the monkey. Call out three names of children who are to line up to give a banana to the monkey. Ask the children, 'Put your hand up if you are last.' The children swap places and you repeat the activity.	• A real or toy banana					
4 Recap. What did we do **first**? What did we do **next**? What did we do **last**? Show items to give prompts.						

Follow-on classroom activity
When the children are lining up, explain that the last person has to look after the line. Use the sign and symbol for 'last' and ask the children 'Who is last in the line?'

Sound Awareness Session Sheet

Week 8

Learning objectives
- To listen for a sound from a choice of two and respond appropriately
- To identify which words rhyme
- To understand the concept 'middle'

Date:		Names of children and notes on their progress				
Activities	**Resources**					
1 Set out two bricks, each with one of the letters 'f' and 'b' next to it. Each child listens for one of the sounds and then adds a brick to the correct tower.	• Letters 'f' and 'b' • Bricks that can be built into a tower					
2 Explain that you are going to say two words. The child has to tell you whether they rhyme or sound alike. Use different words from last week: eg 'pot' and 'dot', 'cup' and 'dog'. Ask the child to point to the yes/no or happy/sad face.	• Template 45: Yes/no or happy/sad faces					
3 Introduce the concept '**middle**' using the sign and symbol. The children pretend to line up for some sweets. Ask the children to 'Put up your hand if you are in the middle.'						
4 Recap. What did we do **first**? What did we do **next**? What did we do **last**? Show items to give prompts.						

Follow-on classroom activity
During carpet time, the children have to listen for their name and then to go to their table or collect their coat.
Explain that you will say some silly words and if it rhymes with their name, they can go.

Sound Awareness Session Sheet

Week 9

Learning objectives
- To listen for a sound and respond appropriately
- To identify which words rhyme
- To understand the concept 'middle'

Date:

Activities	Resources	Names of children and notes on their progress				
1 Give each child a letter of the alphabet and tell them the sound it makes. When each child hears his sound, he holds up the letter.	• Separate alphabet letters					
2 Explain that you are going to say a word and that the child is to say which other words rhyme with it, eg 'Which word rhymes with "house" – "doll" or "mouse"?' If the child has difficulty with this, say two words and ask for a yes/no response to whether they rhyme or not.	• Template 46: Rhyme sheet (List 1) • To help with remembering, use three different-coloured counters to point to as you say each word. Keep the first counter for the first word separate from the other two					
3 Tell the children that you are going to think about the '**middle**'. Three children line up to hang some clothes on the washing line. The adult asks the child in the middle to hold up his article of clothing. Ask the children to swap places and repeat.	• At least three items of clothing, clothes pegs and a washing line, if available					
4 Recap. What did we do **first**? What did we do **next**? What did we do **last**? Show items to give prompts.						

Follow-on classroom activity
During carpet time, as you call out each child's name, ask them to say a word that rhymes with their name. If this is difficult, give the first sound, eg Ali, bee. Or give a choice or two words, one of which rhymes with their name, eg 'Does Dake or Nop rhyme with Jake?'

Week 10

Sound Awareness Session Sheet

Learning objectives
- To listen for a sound and respond appropriately
- To understand the concept and label for 'word'
- To identify which words rhyme

Date:

Activities	Resources	Names of children and notes on their progress			
1 Give each child a letter of the alphabet and tell the child the sound it makes. When each child hears his sound, he jumps into the hoop.	• Separate alphabet letters • A hoop				
2 Each child identifies the word that rhymes with the one you say, for example, "Which word rhymes with "tap" – "cap" or "coat"?' If the children are able, ask them to choose from three words rather than two.	• Template 46: Rhyme sheet with lists of two words (List 1) and three words (List 2)				
3 Tell the children that, together, you are going to think about words. Talk about how words tell us things. 'Go' tells us to do something and 'cat' tells us what something is. Look at a book and point to some words. Show the children the gaps between the words. Each child has to find a word on the page. Tell each child that they have to listen for the word 'go' and then they can put the toy down the tube.	• A book with some large print • A cardboard tube • A toy that will fit into the tube easily				
4 Recap. What did we do **first**? What did we do **next**? What did we do **last**? Show items to give prompts.					

Follow-on classroom activity
Ask the children to find some words in a book they are looking at. Can they point to each word or count the words?

Sound Awareness Session Sheet

Week 11

Learning objectives
- To correctly identify the named word from two that sound similar
- To give an example of a word that rhymes
- To move a counter for each word

Date:

Activities	Resources	Names of children and notes on their progress				
1 All the children share a single lotto board, on which each pair of words has one different sound (eg 'tea' / 'key'). You name one of the items shown and the child has to find the picture of it on the board.	• Template 47: Lotto board (4)					
2 Read aloud a sentence from the sheet. Each child has to complete the sentence with the rhyming word when you give the initial sound.	• Template 48: Rhyme and riddle completion (part 1)					
3 Remind the children about listening for a word. Today they have to listen for words and move a spot or counter heard for each word. You say one word to each child, asking him to repeat the word as he moves the spot or counter. Use one– and then two-syllable words.	• Template 49: Word lists (parts 1 and 2) • Counters, or spots to stick on a Velcro® board					
4 Recap. What did we do **first**? What did we do **next**? What did we do **last**? Show items to give prompts.						

Follow-on classroom activity
During circle time, the teacher whispers a word to one child who whispers it to the next child. This goes all the way around the circle and the last child says the word aloud.

Sound Awareness Session Sheet

Week 12

Learning objectives
- To correctly identify the named word from two that sound similar
- To move a counter for each word
- To give an example of a word that rhymes

Date:		Names of children and notes on their progress			
Activities	**Resources**				
1 All of the children share a single lotto board, on which each pair of words has one different sound. Tell the children that the pictures illustrate the words: 'sit', 'sick', 'hit', 'hid', 'case', 'Kate', 'bow', 'boat'. You name one of the words illustrated and the child has to find it on the board.	• Template 50: Lotto board (5)				
2 Using Template 48, read a riddle to each child and ask him to complete the last word.	• Template 48: Rhyme and riddle completion (part 2)				
3 You say two words to each child. He moves a spot or counter as he repeats each word. You should demonstrate this first.	• Template 49: Word lists (part 3) • Counters, or spots to stick on a Velcro® board				
4 Recap. What did we do **first**? What did we do **next**? What did we do **last**? Show items to give prompts.					

Follow-on classroom activity
During story time, read a storybook with text that rhymes. Suggested books are *Room on the Broom, The Gruffalo, The Cat in the Hat*, etc.

Sound Awareness Session Sheet

Week 13

Learning objectives
- To listen carefully to other people
- To identify which words rhyme
- To move a counter for each word

Date:

Activities	Resources	Names of children and notes on their progress				
1 The children stand in a line. The first child comes to you, and you whisper an instruction for an action. The child then whispers this to the next child, and so on until it reaches the last child. This person must run to the front and do the action. The whisper cannot be repeated, so the children must listen carefully.	• Example of action instructions whispered: 'Clap three times', 'Jump and then wave', 'Touch your toes, point to your nose, then your ears' • Use no more than two instructions if a child has difficulty remembering sequences					
2 Using the picture materials, select one picture to show the child. Place two other pictures in front of the child (one of which rhymes with the target picture). Ask the child to find a picture that rhymes with the one you are holding.	• Template 51: Rhyme pictures (1) cut out to make separate cards; intended rhyme pairs are star/car, house/mouse, light/fight, hop/mop. Use one of the following as a distractor: fish/bag/sweet/ten • Template 52: Rhyme pictures (2); intended rhyme pictures are tree/bee, boat/coat, tea/key, dog/frog (cut out to make separate cards) • Scissors					
3 You say two words and the child moves the counters as he repeats each word.	• Counters, or spots on a Velcro® board • Template 53: Lists of words and phrases (part 1)					
4 Recap. What did we do **first**? What did we do **next**? What did we do **last**? Show items to give prompts.						

Follow-on classroom activity
During story time, read a storybook with text that rhymes. Omit some endings and see whether the children can supply the missing word. Suggested books are *Room on the Broom*, *The Gruffalo*, *The Cat in the Hat*, etc.

Sound Awareness Session Sheet

Week 14

Learning objectives

- To listen carefully to other people
- To identify which words rhyme
- To move a counter for each word

Date:

Activities	Resources	Names of children and notes on their progress				
1 Child A stands in the middle of a circle, blindfolded. The other children are seated in the circle. Child A turns around, stops and points to a child. That child must say 'Hello – guess who I am!' Child A guesses and, if correct, they swap places. If not correct, child A has one more turn. To make it more difficult, the children can try to disguise their voices.	• A suitable blindfold					
2 Show each child three pictures and invite the child to find the two that rhyme with each other. If the child has difficulty, point to one of the pictures that rhyme and see if he can find the one that rhymes with it.	• Templates 51 and 52: Rhyme pictures (1) and (2) cut out to make separate cards • Scissors					
3 You say to each child one three-word phrase. The child moves the counters as he repeats each word.	• Template 53: Lists of words and phrases (part 2) • Counters, or spots to stick on a Velcro® board					
4 Recap. What did we do **first**? What did we do **next**? What did we do **last**? Show items to give prompts.						

Follow-on classroom activity

Activity 1 from the group: child A stands in the middle of a circle, blindfolded. The other children are seated in the circle. Child A turns around, stops and points to a child. That child must say, 'Hello – guess who I am!' Child A guesses and, if correct, they swap places. If not correct, child A has one more turn.

Sound Awareness Session Sheet

Week 15

Learning objectives
- To listen for a word in a story
- To identify which words rhyme
- To identify the first and last words from a list of three

Date:

Activities	Resources	Names of children and notes on their progress				
1 Explain that you are going to read a story. When the children hear the word 'cat' they have to make a 'miaow' sound.	• Template 54: Cat story					
2 Present the child with three pictures, two of which rhyme and one which does not. Ask the child to find the two pictures that rhyme. If he has difficulty, point to one of the rhyming pictures and ask him to find the one that rhymes with it.	• Templates 55 and 56: Rhyme pictures (3) and (4) cut out to make separate cards • Scissors					
3 Tell the children they have to listen for the **'first'** word in a group of three that you are about to say to them. Say the three words, pointing to a different spot for each word, going from the child's left to right. Ask each child to tell you the first word you said. Repeat this activity asking the children to listen for the **'last'** word. Show the last section of the train and again point to the appropriate spot as you say each word.	• Template 53: Lists of words and phrases (parts 3 and 4) • Template 59: Train • Three counters, or spots to stick on a Velcro® board to represent each word					
4 Recap. What did we do **first**? What did we do **next**? What did we do **last**? Show items to give prompts.						

Follow-on classroom activity

For each part of the day use the sign and symbol 'first' and 'last' to tell the children what they are going to do. Draw a picture of what the first, next and last activities will be next to the symbols.

This may be a picture of a book for story time, for example. At the end of the activities, recap by asking the children 'What did we do first today?' Show the children the symbol and the picture next to it to help them recall the activity. Then ask 'What was next?' and 'What did we do last?'

Sound Awareness Session Sheet

Week 16

Learning objectives

- To listen for a word in a story
- To identify which words rhyme
- To identify the last and middle words from a list of three

Date:

Activities	Resources	Names of children and notes on their progress			
1 Before reading a familiar story to the children, warn them that you might make a mistake. If they know what is wrong, they can shout out. Read the story and substitute some of the words or names of some of the characters.	• A familiar story to read aloud				
2 Present four pictures (two sets that rhyme), all muddled up. The child has to identify the rhyming pairs. Word list: 'bow', 'snow', 'pen', 'hen', 'bit', 'sit', 'eye', 'pie', 'car', 'star', 'bed', 'bread', 'house', 'mouse', 'clock', 'sock'.	• Templates 57 and 58: Rhyming picture pairs (1) and (2) (copied and cut out as instructed) • Scissors				
3 Tell the children they have to listen for the **'last'** word in a group of three that you are about to say to them. Show the last part of the train. Say the three words, each time, pointing to a different three for each word, going from the child's left to right. Ask each child to tell you the last word you said. Repeat this activity, asking the children to listen for the **'middle'** word.	• Template 53: Lists of words and phrases (part 3) • Template 59: Train • Counters, or spots to stick on a Velcro® board				
4 Recap. What did we do **first**? What did we do **next**? What did we do **last**? Show items to give prompts.					

Follow-on classroom activity
Table top activity: use pictures of words that rhyme (Templates 57 and 58). Children match the rhyming pairs.

Sound Awareness Session Sheet

Week 17

Learning objectives
- To listen carefully to other people
- To identify which words rhyme
- To identify the first, last and middle words from a list of three

Date:		
		Names of children and notes on their progress
Activities	**Resources**	
1 Sit the children in a circle and tell them that we are going to take turns to say the words 'tick' and 'tock'. The first person says 'tick' and then the next says 'tock', going round the circle. If the children manage this well, explain that you will repeat it but this time if someone says 'clock', the turns go round the other way.		
2 Present four pictures (two sets that rhyme) all muddled up. The child has to find the pairs of pictures that rhyme.	• Templates 57 and 58: Rhyming picture pairs (1) and (2) (copied and cut out) • Scissors	
3 Tell the children that they are going to listen to a list of three words and then they will be asked to repeat one of them. It may be the **first**, **middle** or **last** word, so they must listen very carefully. Point to the counters or spots as you say the words. Use the train to show the child which position word you want them to recall.	• Template 59: Train • Template 53: Lists of words and phrases (part 3) • Counters, or spots to stick on a Velcro® board	
4 Recap. What did we do **first**? What did we do **next**? What did we do **last**? Show items to give prompts.		

Follow-on classroom activity
Play the 'tick, tock' game from Activity 1.

Sound Awareness Session Sheet

Week 18

Learning objectives

- To listen carefully to other people
- To give examples of words that rhyme
- To identify the first, last and middle words from a phrase

Date:		Names of children and notes on their progress				
Activities	**Resources**					
1 Each child holds an item and you call out the names of the different items. When they hear their item called, they hold it up. Start slowly and then speed up as you name the items. To make it more difficult, look at a different child from the one who is holding the item you call out.	• Items to hold. Use topic items where appropriate, eg toy baby animals, small toy model insects for mini-beast topic					
2 Show the children that you can make words rhyme by changing the first sound. Write 'cat' on the board and tell the children what it says. Then rub out the 'c' and add 's', telling them that this now says 'sat': 'cat' and 'sat' rhyme. Continue this with other sounds to make more rhyming words, eg 'hot'/'pot', 'dig'/'pig'. At the end, ask each child to think of a word that rhymes with 'cat'.	• Board and marker pen					
3 Tell the children that they are going to listen to three words in a phrase. They have to tell you one of them. It may be the first, middle or last word. Point to the spots as you say the words. Use the train to show the child which position word you want them to recall.	• Template 53: Lists of words and phrases (part 4) • Template 59: Train • Counters, or spots to stick on a Velcro® board					
4 Recap. What did we do **first**? What did we do **next**? What did we do **last**? Show items to give prompts.						

Follow-on classroom activity

As a warm-up activity, the children listen to you describe something about them or something to wear. If they are wearing it, they stand up: eg 'Stand up if you are wearing white socks.' 'Stand up if you have brown hair.'

Sound Awareness Session Sheet

Week 19

Learning objectives

- To identify familiar sounds
- To give examples of words that rhyme
- To move a counter for each word spoken

Date:

Activities	Resources	Names of children and notes on their progress			
1 Give the children items that make familiar sounds and let the children explore them. Then ask each child in turn to look away while one of their friends makes a sound with one of the items. The child has to listen and guess which item it is.	• Common items that make sounds (eg cup and spoon, pencil and paper, keys, zip on a coat, book)				
2 Show the children that you can make words rhyme by changing the first sound. Write 'van' on the board and tell the children what it says. Then rub out the 'v' and add 'm', telling them that this now says 'man': 'van' and 'man' rhyme. Continue this with other sounds to make more rhyming words. At the end, ask each child to think of a word that rhymes with 'van'.	• Board and marker pen				
3 Explain that you are going to say some words. You want each child to repeat each word and push a counter or spot into a square on the board as they say each word.	• Template 60: Short sentences • Counters and a squared board (board or paper with five squares next to each other), or spots to stick on a Velcro® board				
4 Recap. What did we do **first**? What did we do **next**? What did we do **last**? Show items to give prompts.					

Follow-on classroom activity
Table top activity: draw something that rhymes with 'sat'.

Week 20

Sound Awareness Session Sheet

Learning objectives
- To listen to and follow an instruction
- To give examples of words that rhyme
- To identify and say the separate syllables that make up words

Date:		Names of children and notes on their progress				
Activities	**Resources**					
1 Give each child an instruction to follow. But explain that they cannot do it until you say 'Go'. Give instructions such as 'Touch your nose', 'Wave your hand', 'Stand up', 'Knock on the door', 'Close your eyes'.						
2 Remind the children about rhyming. In a circle, each child takes turns to hold the object (eg a pear) and give an example of a word that rhymes with that object, eg 'bear'. Then they pass the object to the next child. Other words to rhyme: car, hat, pen, bed.	• Items to pass round the circle such as toy car, pear, hat, pen, toy bed					
3 Introduce 'Robot' and tell the children that he talks in a funny way. Demonstrate this by saying the children's names in syllables, eg 'Ni–cho–las', 'Dan–iel'. Can each child recognise his name when you say it like this? Pass the robot round, asking each child to say their own name like the robot would.	• Template 61: Robot					
4 Recap. What did we do **first**? What did we do **next**? What did we do **last**? Show items to give prompts.						

Follow-on classroom activity
Select children (by saying their names in syllables) to collect their coats by saying their name using 'Robot' talking.

Routledge
Taylor & Francis Group

Sound Awareness Session Sheet

Week 21

Learning objectives

- To listen for a sound and respond appropriately
- To give examples of words that rhyme
- To identify and say the separate syllables that make up words

Date:

Activities	Resources	Names of children and notes on their progress				
1 Each child holds the toy animal and has a turn to listen for the noise it makes. You make lots of animal sounds; when the child hears the sound of that particular animal, he pulls it away quickly, as you try to catch it.	• Toy animal					
2 The children stand up and you tell them what word you are thinking about. If the children know a word that rhymes with it, they can jump in the hoop and say their word. Words to rhyme: 'door', 'bow', 'eat', 'cake'.	• Hoop					
3 Introduce 'Robot' and remind the children of how he talks (in syllables). Explain that Robot is going to tell each child which item to post in the box. They listen to you doing the robot talking and find the item to post in the box.	• Template 61: Robot • Items to post in a box (eg scissors, pencil, paper, toy dinosaur, toy elephant) • Box of a suitable size					
4 Recap. What did we do **first**? What did we do **next**? What did we do **last**? Show items to give prompts.						

Follow-on classroom activity

Before the children go out to play, ask them to say a word that rhymes with one you say. This is the secret password to let them go to play! If they have difficulty, give them a choice or tell them the words that rhyme.

Week 22

Sound Awareness Session Sheet

Learning objectives
- To listen to and follow an instruction
- To listen for a sound and respond appropriately
- To identify and say the separate syllables that make up words

Date:

Activities	Resources	Names of children and notes on their progress			
1 Explain that you are going to tell the children to do something if they are wearing certain items. Give an instruction, eg: 'Stand up if you have brown hair', 'Clap your hands if you are wearing black socks'.					
2 Introduce 'Snail', who says sounds. Tell each child they have to listen to lots of sounds but only when they hear a certain target sound do they have to put a counter in the pot. You then make different sounds (eg 'p', 't', 'k', 's', 'f'), including the target sound.	• Template 62: Snail • Counters for each child • A pot to put them in (either one for the entire group, or one pot each)				
3 Cut the picture cards in half. Ask each child to say the word in two parts (eg 'ki-tten'). When each child has had a turn, they then take turns to say it along with the child next to them. Each child should only say one syllable. Pass the picture parts on to the next child so each child has a turn to say the first and last syllable of the word.	• Templates 63 and 64: Two-syllable word pictures (1) and (2) • Template 61: Robot, to remind children about talking in syllables • Scissors				
4 Recap. What did we do **first**? What did we do **next**? What did we do **last**? Show items to give prompts.					

Follow-on classroom activity
During circle time, children take it in turns to say and clap out their name like Robot talking. The adults can demonstrate this. Each child has a go as the turns pass round the circle.

Sound Awareness Session Sheet

Week 23

Learning objectives
- To listen to and follow an instruction
- To listen for a sound in a word and respond appropriately
- To identify and say the separate syllables that make up words

Date:	Resources	Names of children and notes on their progress			
Activities	**Resources**				
1 Give each child an individual instruction to go and get something from the classroom. All of the children have to wait until everybody has been told their own instruction; then, when you say 'Go', they all carry out their instruction.	• A pencil and paper to jot down a reminder of what you have told each child to collect				
2 Explain that Snail is going to say some silly words really slowly. Each child has to listen for the 's' sound in that word and, if they hear it, they can post the toy car down the tube. You say: 'tee', 'kee', 'fee', 'see', 'lee', 'chee', 'see', 'gee', 'see', 'dee', 'zee', 'see'.	• Template 62: Snail • Cardboard tube (eg from a roll of wrapping paper) • Toy car that fits easily into cardboard tube				
3 Cut the picture cards into three sections. Ask each child to say the word in three parts (eg 'e-le-phant'). Then they take turns to say it with two other children. Each child should only say one syllable. Pass the picture parts on to the next child so that each child has a turn to say the first, middle and last syllable of the word.	• Templates 65 and 66: Three-syllable word pictures (1) and (2) • Template 61: Robot • Scissors				
4 Recap. What did we do **first**? What did we do **next**? What did we do **last**? Show items to give prompts.					

Follow-on classroom activity
Using the class topic, select some key words (as pictures) and demonstrate how we can say the words in syllables, talking like Robot. Ask the children to clap and say the key words in syllables.

Sound Awareness Session Sheet

Week 24

Learning objectives
- To listen for a word and respond appropriately
- To listen for a sound in a word and respond appropriately
- To identify and say the separate syllables that make up words

Date:

Activities	Resources	Names of children and notes on their progress				
1 Seat the children so they are alternately facing towards or away from the circle. Each child has a pot and some counters. Call out food items and when they hear 'jelly', they put a counter in their pot. Say a list of words including 'jelly' four times. Ask the children how many counters they have in their pot.	• A pot (or other container) and some counters for each child					
2 Explain that Snail is going to say some silly words really slowly. In turn, each child has to listen for the 'p' sound in that word at the end and, if they hear it, they can throw a beanbag into the hoop. You say: 'ark', 'art', 'arp', 'arf', 'arg', 'arb', 'ard', 'arp', 'arn'.	• Template 62: Snail • One beanbag for each child • One hoop					
3 Explain that, together, you are going to do some more Robot talking. This time each child chooses an item from a bag and claps as they say the word in syllables. Tell the children the words may be one or two claps.	• Template 61: Robot • Items with one- and two-syllable names in an opaque bag (eg car, pencil, book, chicken, apple)					
4 Recap. What did we do **first**? What did we do **next**? What did we do **last**? Show items to give prompts.						

Follow-on classroom activity
Using the class topic, display the key pictures and words on the wall. The title can be 'Can you clap out these words?' Adults can prompt the children to have a go when they are looking at the pictures.

Sound Awareness Session Sheet

Week 25

Learning objectives
- To listen to and repeat a nonsense word
- To blend the sounds of a word together and identify it from individual spoken sounds
- To identify and say the separate syllables that make up words

Date:		Names of children and notes on their progress				
Activities	**Resources**					
1 Explain that each child is going to pretend to be a parrot (show Template 67). Explain that parrots repeat words. Give each child a nonsense word to repeat back.	• Template 67: Parrot • Nonsense words, eg 'fangerpoop', 'shinderbar', 'desoplock', 'tockleduff', 'pufflelop', 'bumblesar'					
2 Place two of the items in the middle of the group. Explain to the children that Frog is going to tell them a word which will be one of the items on the floor. They have to listen carefully and pick up the item. You then say slowly the three sounds in each word (eg 'c … a … t').	• Template 68: Frog • Six items which have names with three sounds each (eg cat, duck, sock, pen, pot, dog)					
3 Explain that, together, you are going to do some more Robot talking. Each child chooses an item from a bag and claps as they say the word in syllables, or moves the counters or spots. Tell the children that the words may be two or three claps long.	• Template 61: Robot • Counters, or spots to stick on a Velcro® board • Toy items with two- and three-syllable names in an opaque bag (eg pencil, ruler, apple, banana, elephant, butterfly)					
4 Recap. What did we do **first**? What did we do **next**? What did we do **last**? Show items to give prompts.						

Follow-on classroom activity
During circle time, play I-Spy but, instead of saying the initial sound, sound out a simple two or three sound word that is visible, eg ch-air, d-oor, p-e-n, c-oa-t, b-i-n, d-o-ll.

Week 26

Sound Awareness Session Sheet

Learning objectives
- To listen to an instruction and carry out actions in the right sequence as part of a group
- To blend the sounds of a word together and identify it from individual spoken sounds
- To identify and say the separate syllables that make up words

Date:

Activities	Resources	Names of children and notes on their progress				
1 Give two children musical instruments to hold. Make sure they know what the instruments are called. Tell them that you will call out the names of the instruments and they must play them in the right order (eg triangle, then drum). Once they can do this, repeat with three children holding three instruments.	• Three musical instruments					
2 Syllable revision: place objects which have names with one, two or three syllables in front of the children. Check that the children know what the items are called. Then tell the children that you are going to clap one item. Can they tell you which one you clapped?	• Six objects with names containing one, two or three syllables (eg chair, soap, pencil, paint brush, elephant, dinosaur)					
3 Introduction to sounds in a word. Place three of the items in the middle of the group. Explain that Frog is going to tell them a word which will be one of the items on the floor. They have to listen carefully and pick up the item. Say the three sounds slowly (eg 'c ... a ... t').	• Template 68: Frog • Six items with names containing three sounds rather than syllables (eg cat, duck, sock, pen, pot, pan)					
4 Recap. What did we do **first**? What did we do **next**? What did we do **last**? Show items to give prompts.						

Follow-on classroom activity
Using the class topic, display the key pictures and words on the wall. The title can be 'Can you clap out these words?' Adults can prompt the children to have a go when they are looking at the pictures.

Sound Awareness Session Sheet

Week 27

Learning objectives
- To listen and respond appropriately to a word
- To blend the sounds of a word together and identify it from individual spoken sounds
- To identify the first sound in a word

Date:

Activities	Resources	Names of children and notes on their progress				
1 Give each child an object to hold. When you call out the names of two objects, the children holding them have to swap places. To make it more difficult, add an extra word (eg 'a *shiny* counter', 'a *blue* book').	• Objects to hold, taken from the classroom (such as red book, blue book, green counter, shiny mirror, big doll, fast car, pretty flower)					
2 Show Snail and tell the children he will choose someone to have a turn at the game. Remind them that he will say their name very slowly, separating the sounds. They have to listen carefully and take their turn when he says their name.	• Template 62: Snail • A fun game such as the marble run or fishing game					
3 Show the children two pictures, each showing objects with names containing two sounds. Pointing to the first part of the train (cover the last carriage), show the children that we are going to listen to the first sound. Say the sounds slowly as you point to each part of the train, then ask which one has '[say sound]' **first** or at the beginning. Can the child find the correct picture?	• Template 59: Train • Sign and symbol 'first' • Template 69: Two-sound word pictures (copied and cut out to make separate cards) • Scissors					
4 Recap. What did we do **first**? What did we do **next**? What did we do **last**? Show items to give prompts.						

Follow-on classroom activity
Before the children go out to play, ask them to listen carefully for their name. Using Snail talk, say each sound in their name slowly, eg K-a-t-y.

Sound Awareness Session Sheet

Week 28

Learning objectives

- To listen to and copy a rhythm
- To identify the first sound in a word
- To blend and segment the sounds of a short word

Date:		Names of children and notes on their progress						
Activities	**Resources**							
1 You clap a rhythm and all the children copy it together. Then each child has his own turn.								
2 Show Snail and tell the children they are going to talk slowly like him. They have to say the name of an item slowly for the next child to find. When the child finds the item, it is his turn.	• Template 62: Snail • Template 70: Three-sound word pictures							
3 Show the children two pictures, each with three sounds. Pointing to the first part of the train, show the children that you are going to listen to the first sound together. Say the sounds slowly as you point to each part of the train. Then ask which one has '[say the sound]' **first** or at the beginning. Can the child find the correct picture?	• Template 59: Train • Sign and symbol 'first' • Template 70: Three-sound word pictures (cut out to make separate cards) • Scissors							
4 Recap. What did we do **first**? What did we do **next**? What did we do **last**? Show items to give prompts.								

Follow-on classroom activity

Table top activity: place items on the table, some of which begin with a target sound, eg 'p'. Children select the items that have 'p' at the beginning and place them in a hoop or circle. Stick the target letter sound onto the hoop or circle.

Sound Awareness Session Sheet

Week 29

Learning objectives

- To listen to and respond appropriately to a sound
- To say the two sounds in a nonsense word
- To identify the last sound in a word

Date:

Activities	Resources	Names of children and notes on their progress			
1 The children pass a hat round the circle and when they hear the bell, the child holding the hat has to put it on.	• Hat • Bell or other percussion instrument				
2 Tell the children that you are going to say a silly word, and you want them to use the spots and tell you what two sounds they heard. Demonstrate this first (eg say 'ar ... p'; then move a spot as you say 'ar', then the next spot as you say 'p').	• Silly words: 'oot', 'eef', 'ock', 'ip', 'foo', 'ke', 'sar', 'gee', 'gar', 'ard' • Counters, or spots to stick on a Velcro® board				
3 Show the children two pictures of objects with names containing three sounds. Pointing to the **last** part of the train, show the children that you are going to listen to the last sound together. Say the sounds slowly as you point to each part of the train, then ask which one has '[say the sound]' last. Can the child find the correct picture?	• Template 59: Train • Sign and symbol 'last' • Template 70: Three-sound word pictures (copied and cut out to make separate cards) • Scissors				
4 Recap. What did we do **first**? What did we do **next**? What did we do **last**? Show items to give prompts.					

Follow-on classroom activity

Circle time activity: the children pass a hat round the circle and, when they hear the bell, the child holding the hat has to put it on.

Week 30

Sound Awareness Session Sheet

Learning objectives
- To listen to and follow an instruction
- To say the two sounds in a nonsense word
- To identify the middle sound in a word

Date:					
Activities	**Resources**	**Names of children and notes on their progress**			
1 Give each child an instruction to follow. Explain that they cannot do it until you say 'Go'. Give instructions such as: 'Touch your nose', 'Wave your hand', 'Stand up', 'Knock on the door', 'Close your eyes'.					
2 Tell the children that you are going to say a silly word, and you want them to use the spots and tell you what two sounds they heard. Demonstrate this first (eg say 'ar ... p'; then move a spot as you say 'ar', then the next spot as you say 'p').	• Counters, or spots to stick on a Velcro® board • Silly words: 'oot', 'eef', 'ock', 'ip', 'foo', 'ke', 'sar', 'gee', 'mar', 'ard'				
3 Show the children two pictures of objects with names containing three sounds. Pointing to the **middle** part of the train, show the children that you are going to listen to the middle sound together. Say the sounds slowly as you point to each part of the train, then ask which one has 'Isay the sound]' in the middle. Can the child find the correct picture?	• Template 59: Train • Sign and symbol 'middle' • Template 70: Three-sound word pictures (copied and cut out to make separate cards) • Scissors				
4 Recap. What did we do **first**? What did we do **next**? What did we do **last**? Show items to give prompts.					

Follow-on classroom activity
Table top activity: place items on the table, some of which have the target sound, eg 'oo', in the middle. Children select the items that have 'oo' in the middle and place them in a hoop or circle. Stick the target letter sound onto the hoop or circle. Items could be pictures of moon, spoon, food, boot, root, and others with a different middle sound.

Part 3

Resource Templates

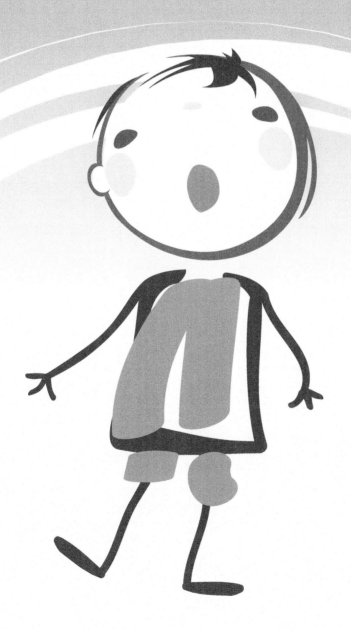

List of Resource Templates

Language templates

Template number	Template title	Weeks used	Home Sheet	Available in colour
1	Lotto board (1)	1, 22, 29		✓
2	Yes/no cards	3		
3	Big and little	3	✓	
4	Food	4, 13, 21		✓
5	Animals (1)	5	✓	
6	Christmas	5, 6	✓	
7	Which pictures are the same?	6	✓	
8	Furniture	7		✓
9	More furniture	7	✓	
10	More food	7, 13, 21		✓
11	Body parts	8	✓	
12	Kitchenware	9	✓	
13	Is it a toy or not?	10	✓	
14	Clothes	11, 15	✓	✓
15	Parts of a house	13	✓	
16	Three sized bears	13, 14	✓	
17	Actions (1)	16, 17, 20		✓
18	Light sources	14	✓	
19	Singular/plural lotto	14		✓
20	Boy and girl	15	✓	
21	Actions (2)	16, 17, 20		✓
22	Fruit	17	✓	
23	Missing parts	18		✓
24	Vegetables	17, 19	✓	
25	Lotto board (2)	7, 19, 22		✓
26	Tools	20	✓	
27	Actions (3)	20		✓
28	Baby animals	21, 24	✓	
29	Shapes	22	✓	
30	Lotto board (3)	22		✓
31	Animals (2)	23		✓
32	The farm	25	✓	✓
33	Category cards (1)	25		✓
34	Parts of a tree	26	✓	✓
35	Happy/sad cards	26, 27		✓
36	Parts of a plant	27	✓	
37	Description clues	27		
38	Seaside	28	✓	✓
39	Category cards (2)	28		✓
40	Picture pairs (1)	28		✓
41	Picture pairs (2)	28		✓
42	Clothes for a hot day	29	✓	
43	Clothes for a cold day	29	✓	
44	Parts of your body	30	✓	

Sound Awareness templates

Template number	Template title	Weeks used	Available in colour
45	Yes/no/happy/sad faces	7, 8	
46	Rhyme sheet	9, 10	
47	Lotto board (4)	11	✓
48	Rhyme and riddle completion	11, 12	
49	Word lists	11, 12	
50	Lotto board (5)	12	✓
51	Rhyme pictures (1)	13, 14	✓
52	Rhyme pictures (2)	13, 14	✓
53	Lists of words and phrases	13, 14, 15, 16, 17, 18	
54	Cat story	15	
55	Rhyme pictures (3)	15	✓
56	Rhyme pictures (4)	15	✓
57	Rhyming picture pairs (1)	16, 17	✓
58	Rhyming picture pairs (2)	16, 17	✓
59	Train	15, 16, 17, 18, 27, 28, 29, 30	✓
60	Short sentences	19	
61	Robot	20, 21, 22, 23, 24, 25	✓
62	Snail	22, 23, 24, 27, 28	✓
63	Two-syllable word pictures (1)	22	✓
64	Two-syllable word pictures (2)	22	✓
65	Three-syllable word pictures (1)	23	✓
66	Three-syllable word pictures (2)	23	✓
67	Parrot	25	✓
68	Frog	25, 26	✓
69	Two-sound word pictures	27	✓
70	Three-sound word pictures	28, 29, 30	✓

Language Templates
1–44

1 Lotto board (1)

Language **Weeks 1, 22, 29**

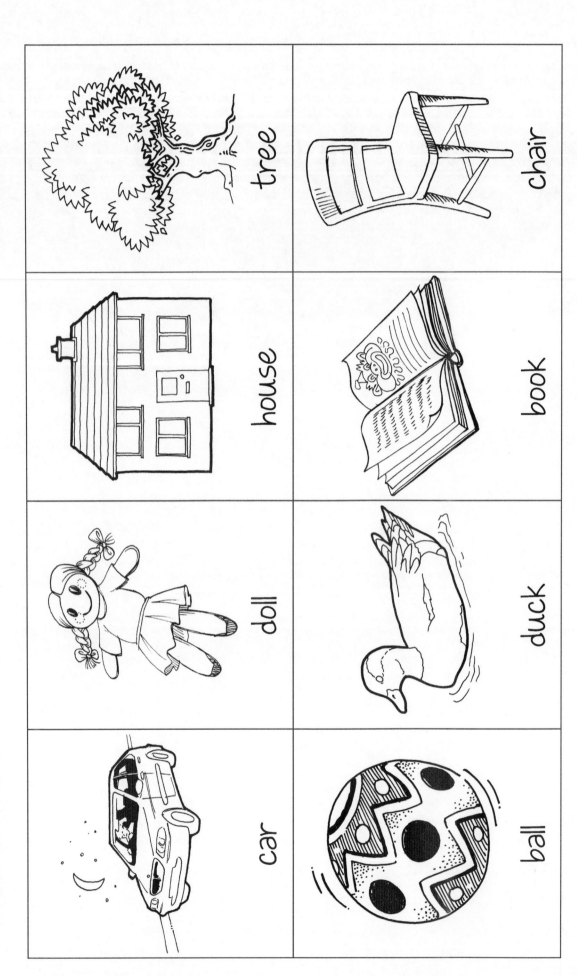

tree

chair

house

book

doll

duck

car

ball

Language **Week 3**

2 **Yes/no cards**

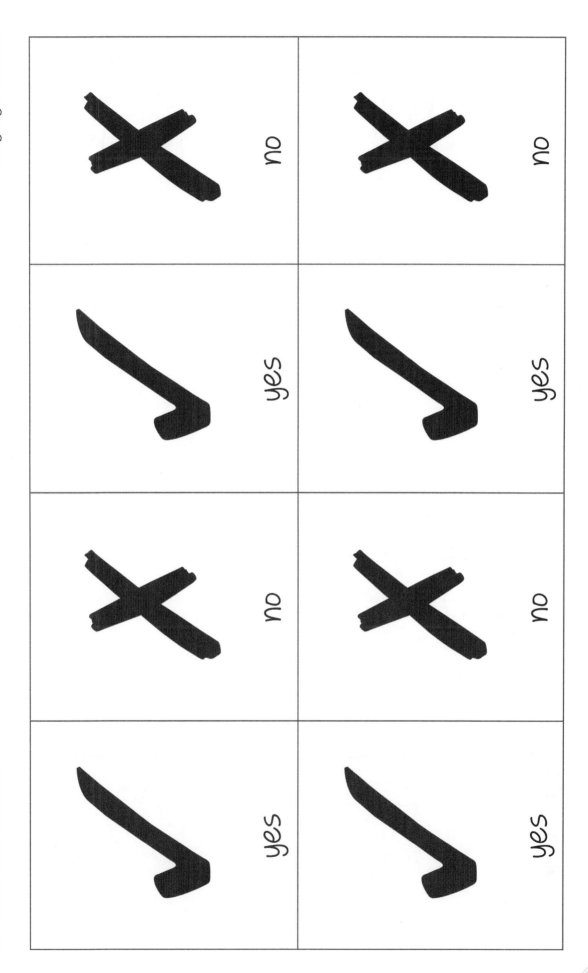

Language **Week 3**

Colour in all the big pictures.

3 **Big and little** 🏠

Language **Weeks 4, 13, 21**

4 **Food**

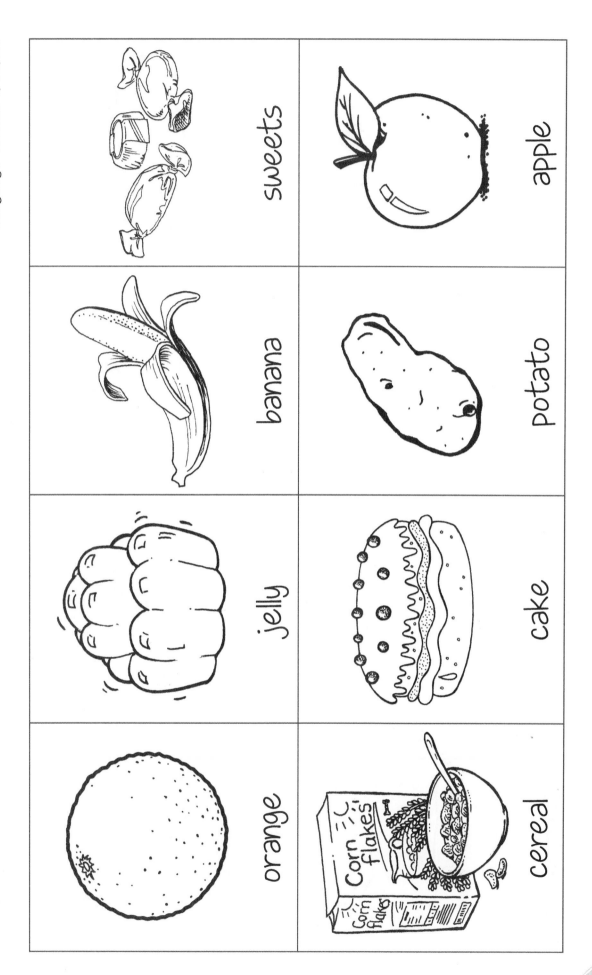

sweets

apple

banana

potato

jelly

cake

orange

cereal

5 **Animals (1)**

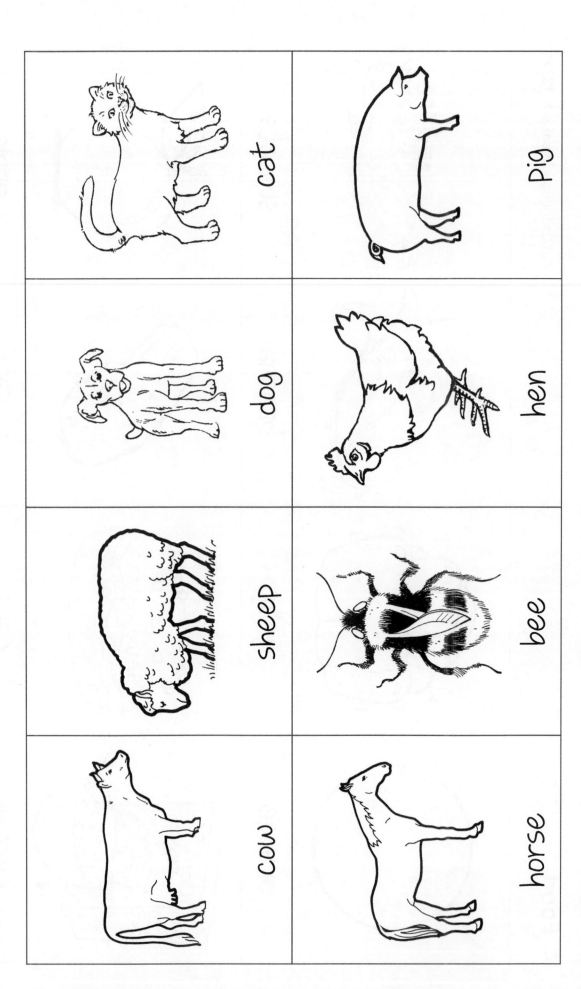

cat

pig

dog

hen

sheep

bee

cow

horse

6 **Christmas**

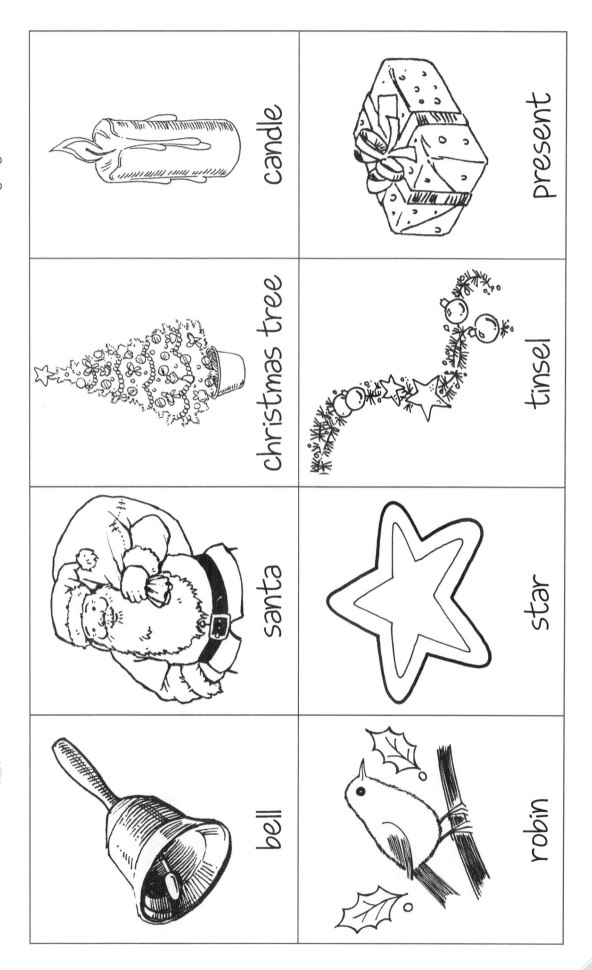

candle

present

christmas tree

tinsel

santa

star

bell

robin

Routledge
Taylor & Francis Group

7 **Which pictures are the same?**

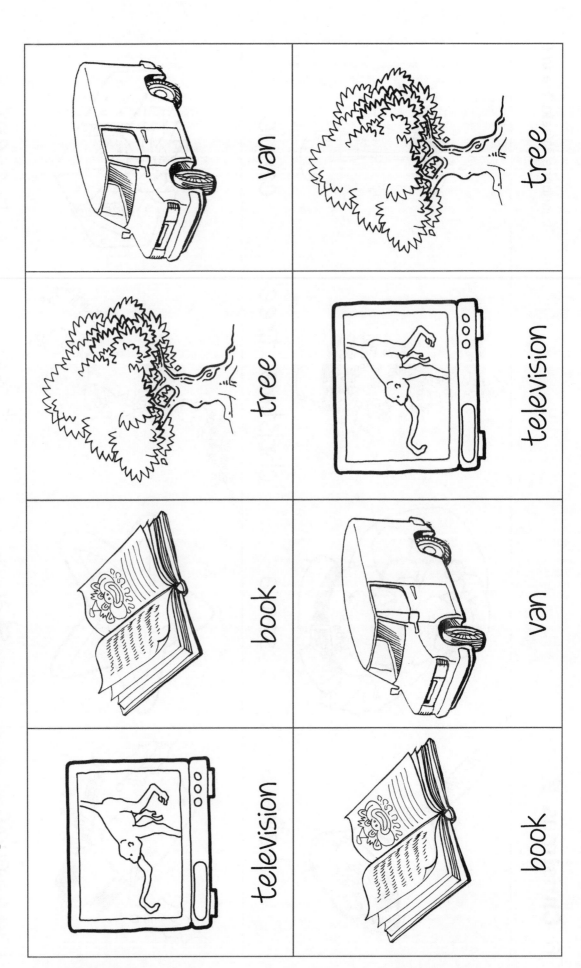

van

tree

tree

television

book

van

television

book

Language **Week 7**

8 **Furniture**

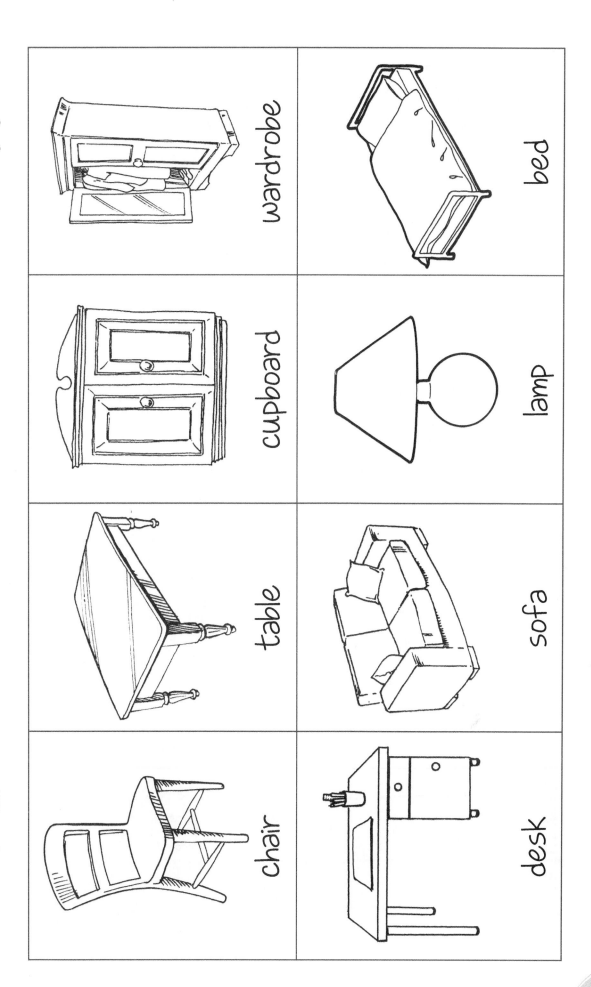

wardrobe

bed

cupboard

lamp

table

sofa

chair

desk

Language **Week 7**

9 **More furniture**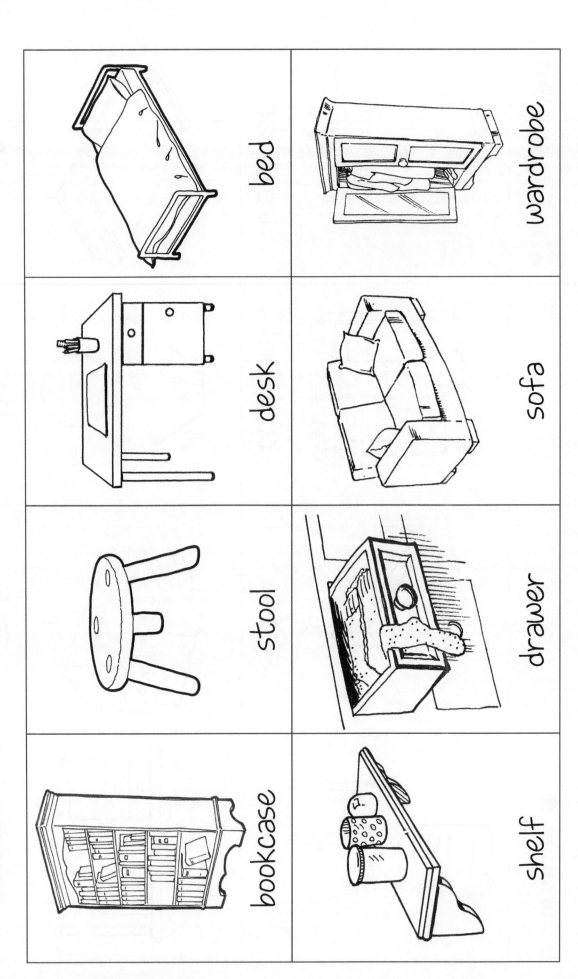

bed

wardrobe

desk

sofa

stool

drawer

bookcase

shelf

10 **More food**

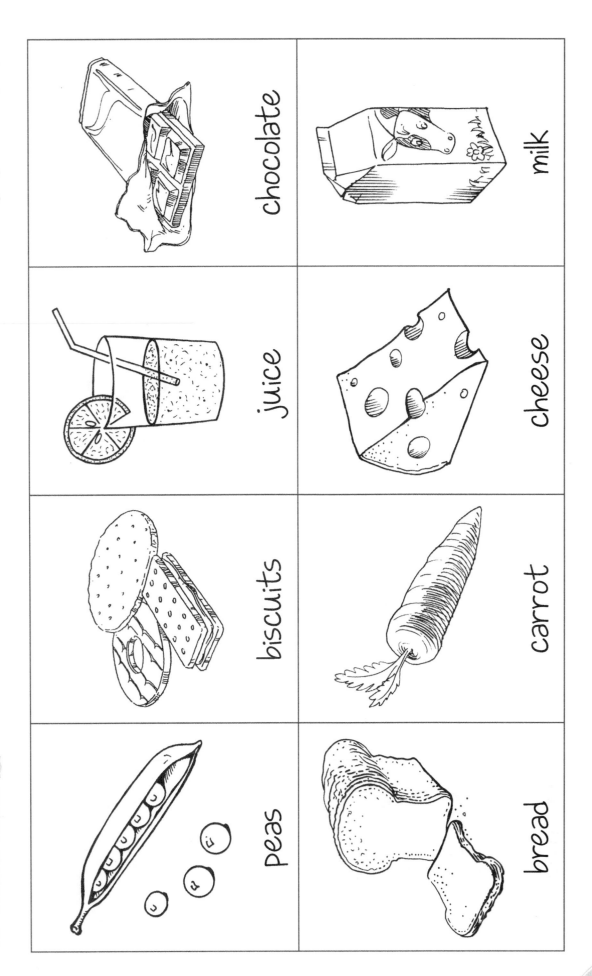

chocolate

milk

juice

cheese

biscuits

carrot

peas

bread

Routledge
Taylor & Francis Group

Language **Week 8**

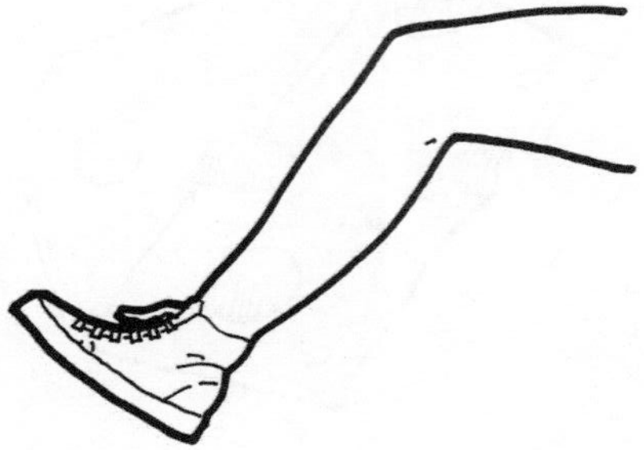

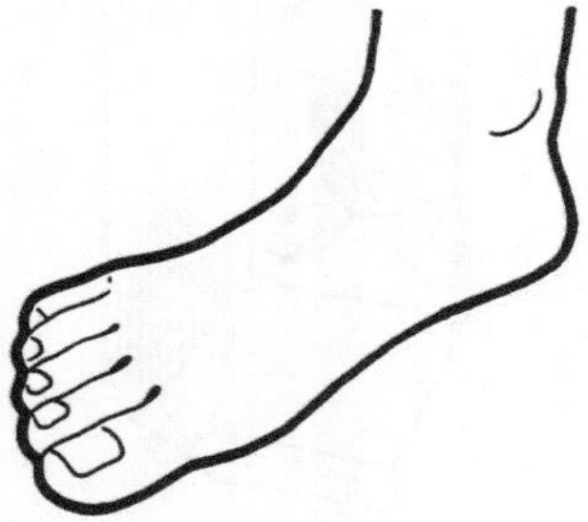

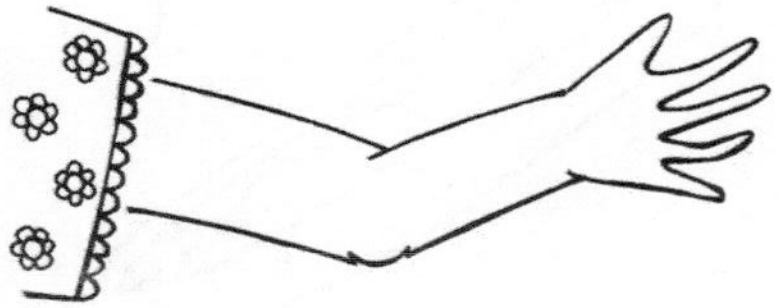

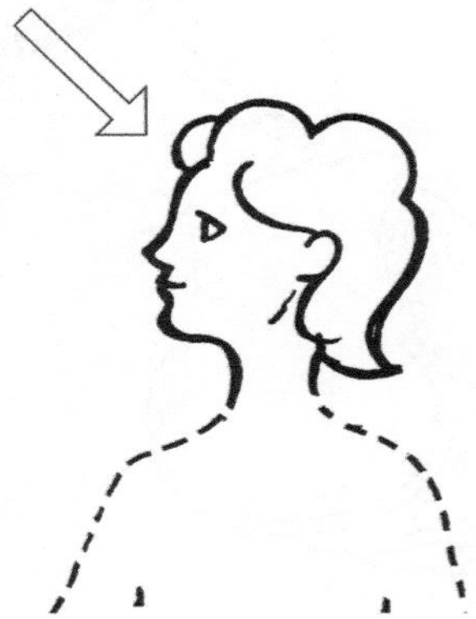

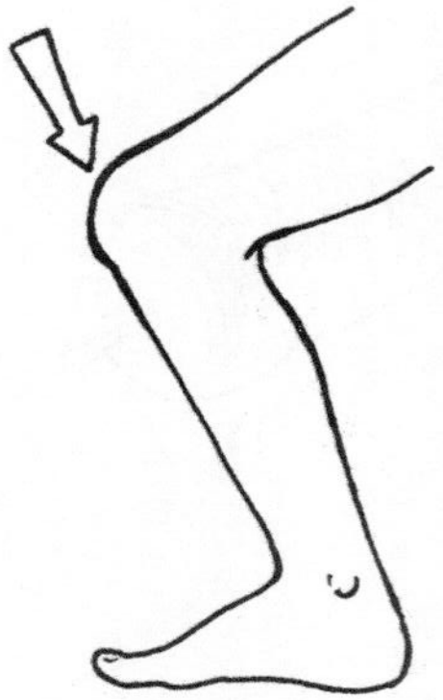

11 **Body parts**

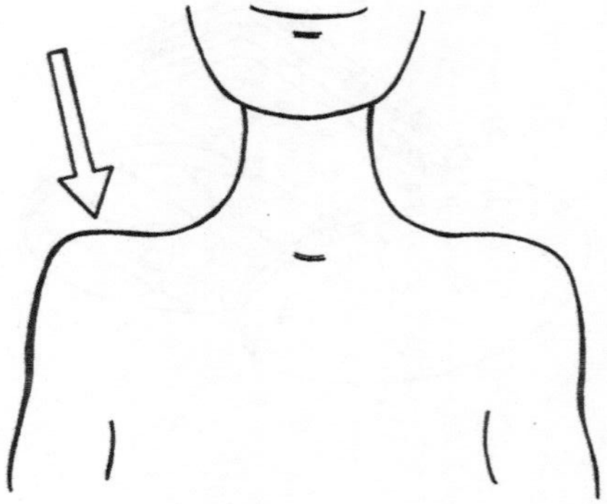

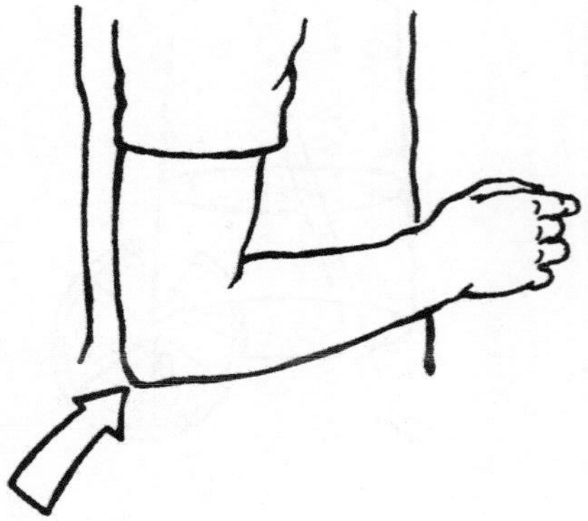

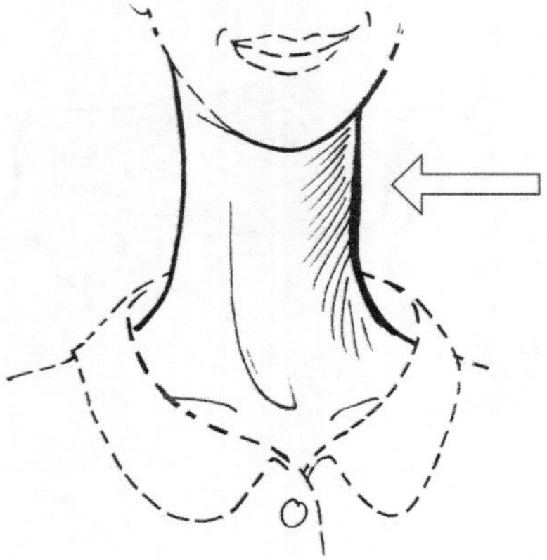

foot

neck

leg

elbow

knee

shoulder

head

arm

Language **Week 9**

12 **Kichenware**

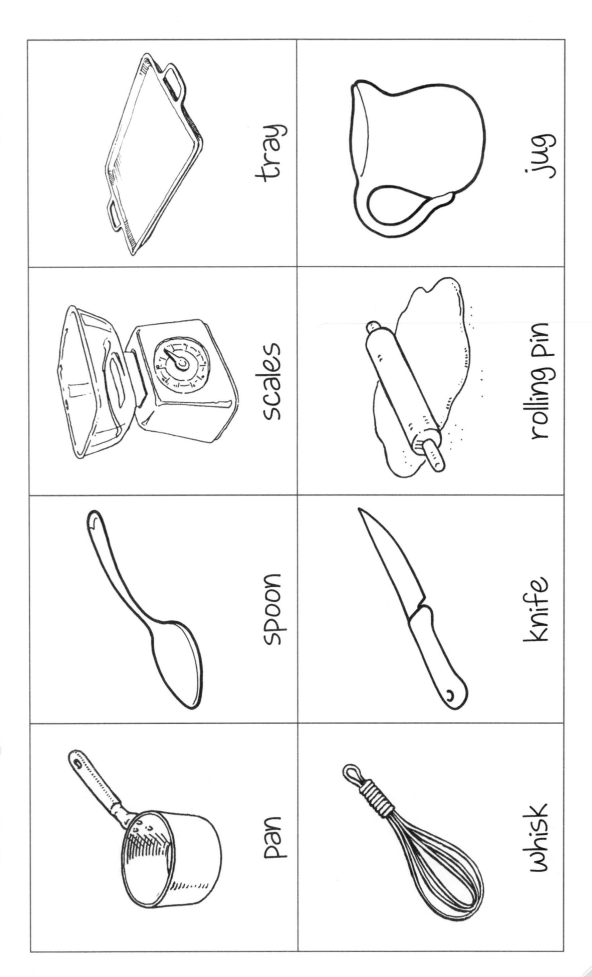

tray

jug

scales

rolling pin

spoon

knife

pan

whisk

Language **Week 10**

Colour in the toys only.

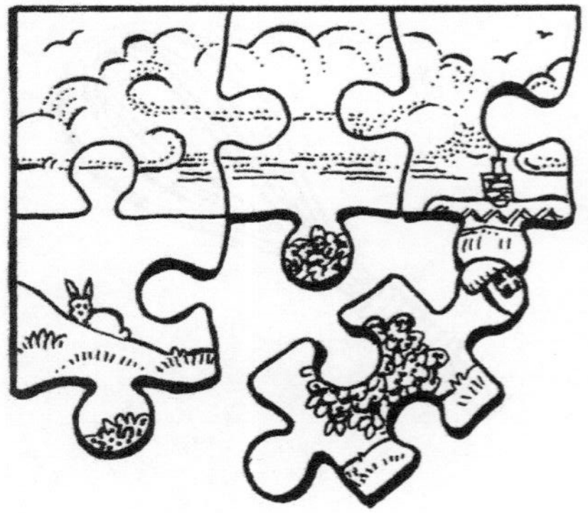

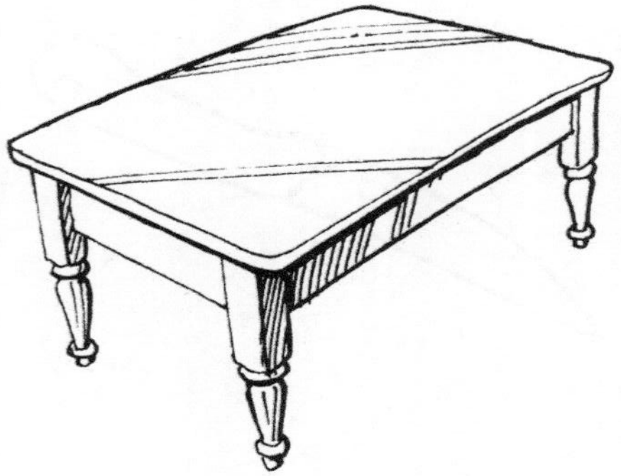

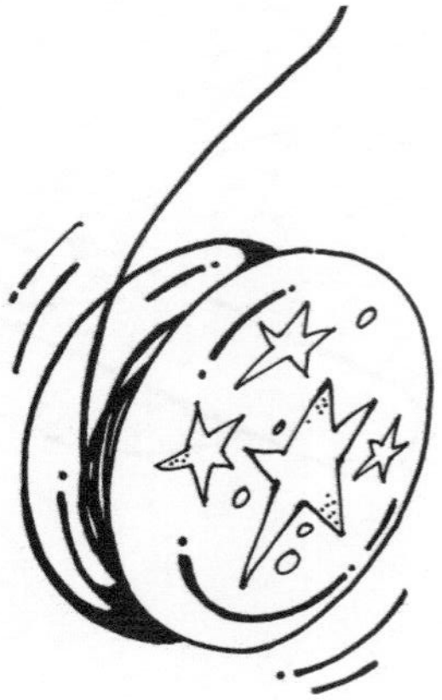

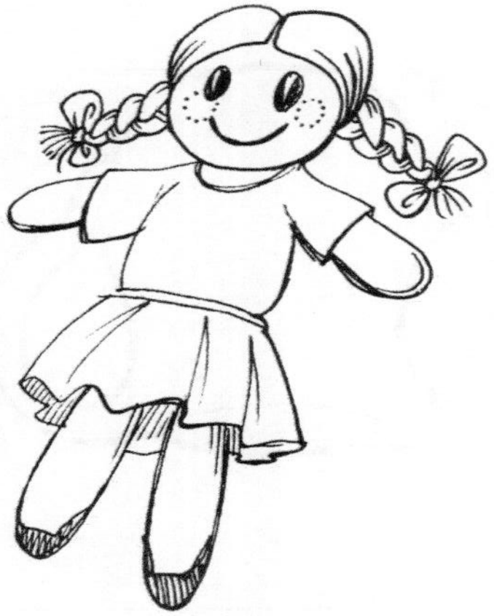

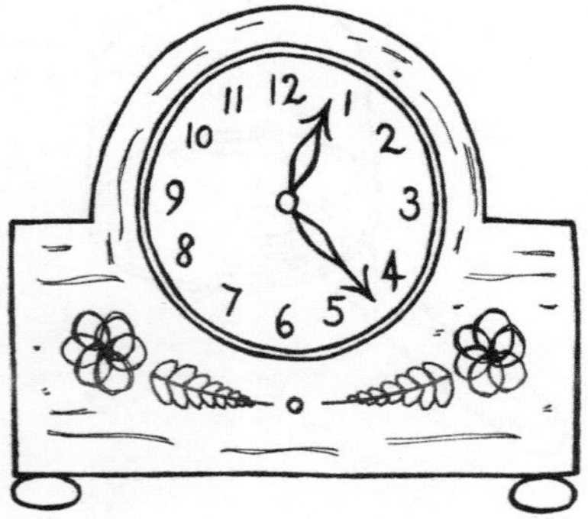

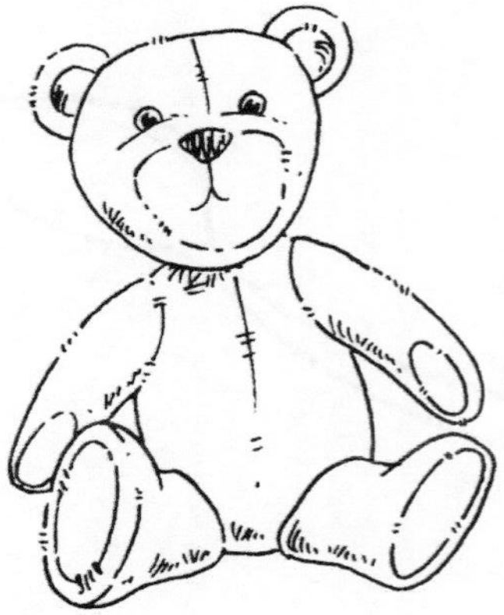

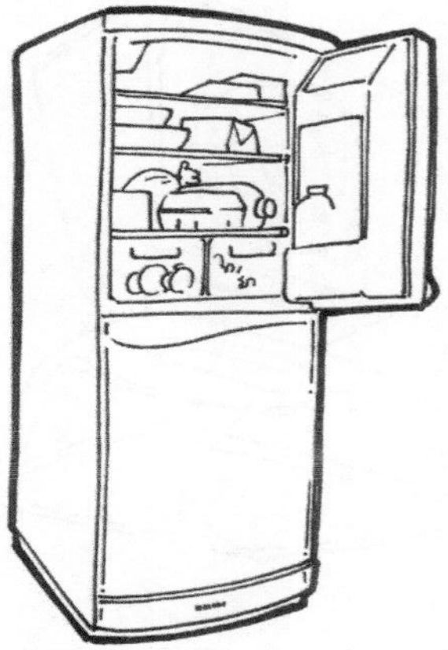

13 Is it a toy or not?

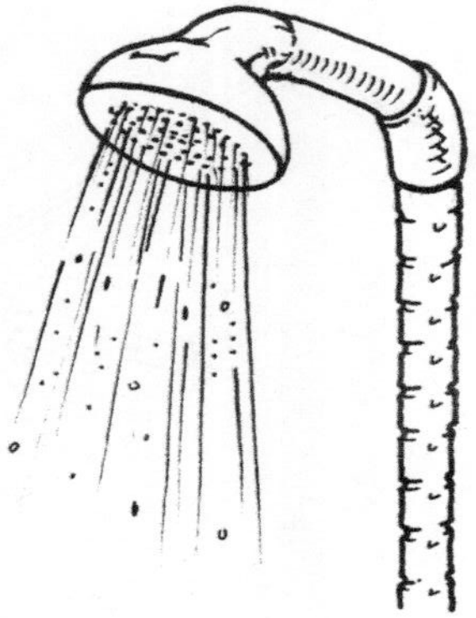

doll

shower

yoyo

fridge

table

teddy

puzzle

clock

14 **Clothes**

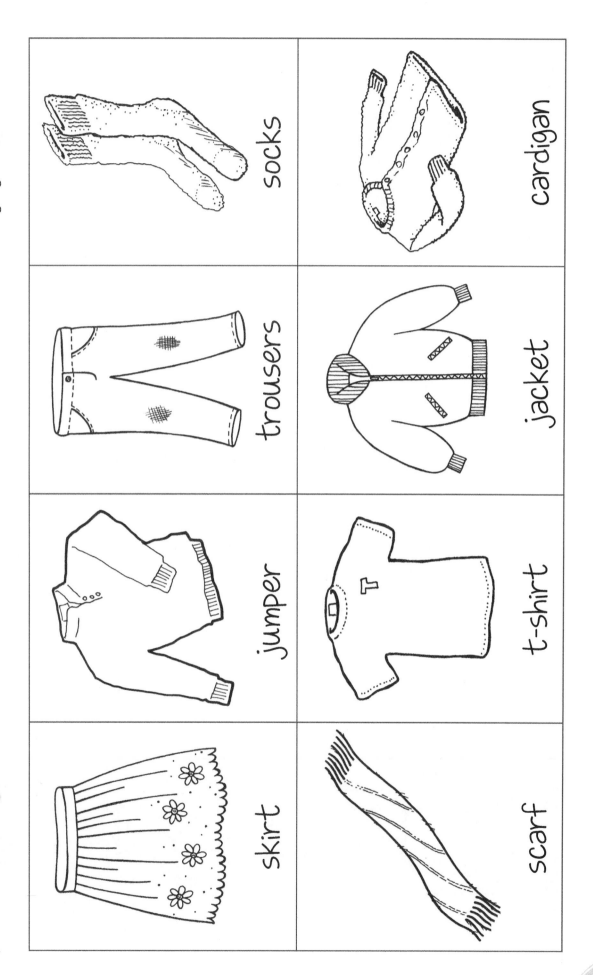

socks

cardigan

trousers

jacket

jumper

t-shirt

skirt

scarf

15 **Parts of a house**

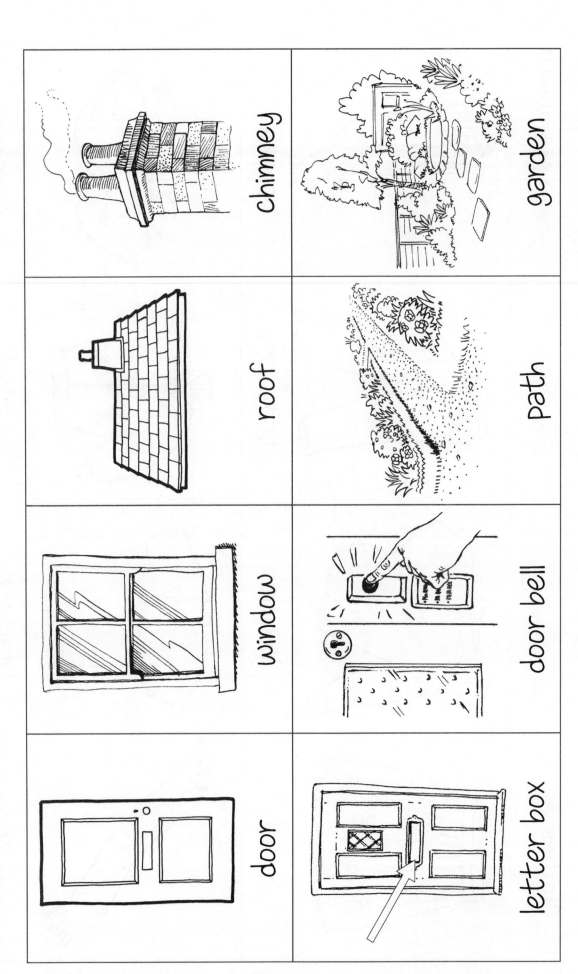

chimney

garden

roof

path

window

door bell

door

letter box

16 **Three sized bears**

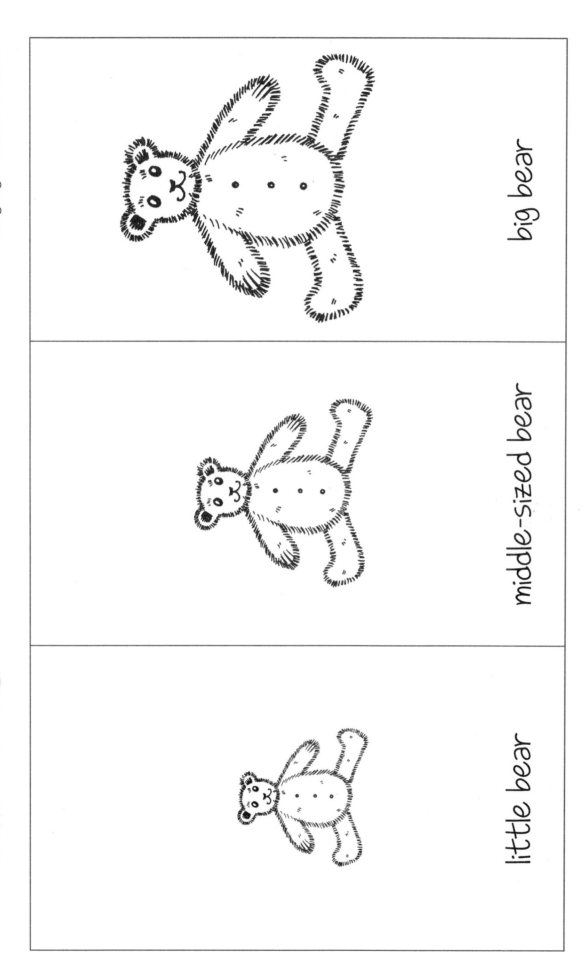

big bear

middle-sized bear

little bear

Routledge
Taylor & Francis Group

Language **Weeks 16, 17, 20**

17 Actions (1)

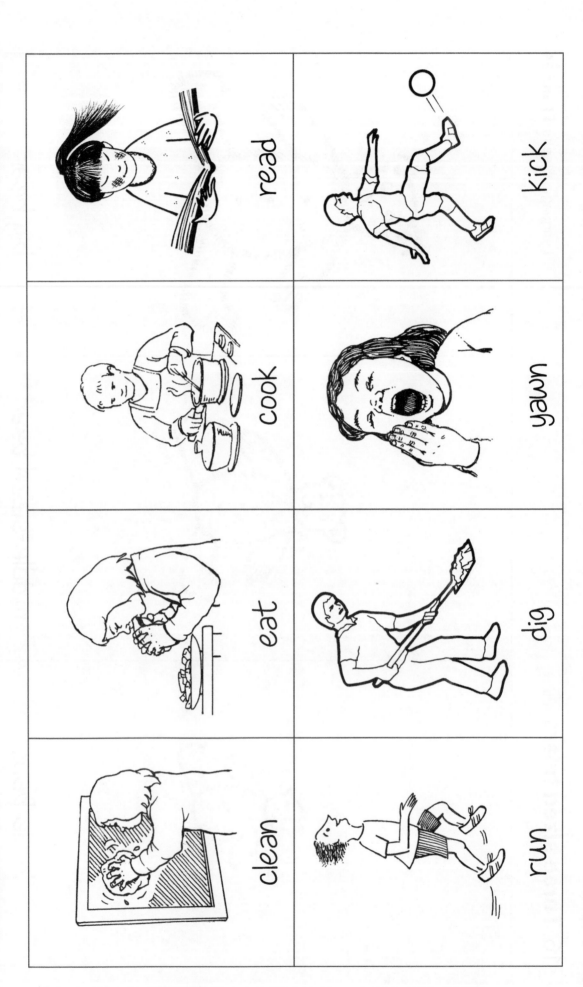

read

kick

cook

yawn

eat

dig

clean

run

18 **Light sources**

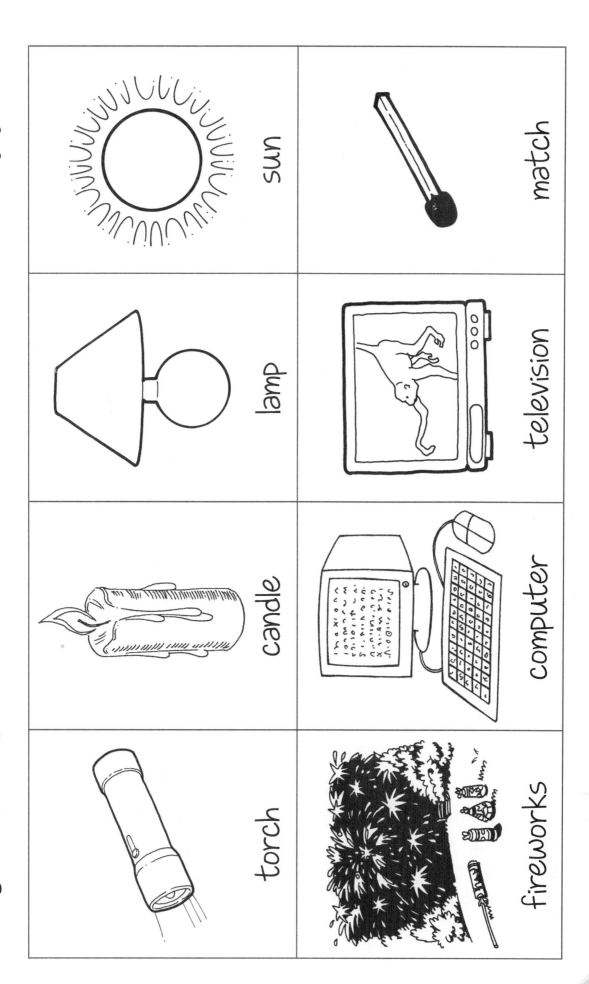

sun

match

lamp

television

candle

computer

torch

fireworks

Routledge
Taylor & Francis Group

Language **Week 14**

19 Singular/plural lotto

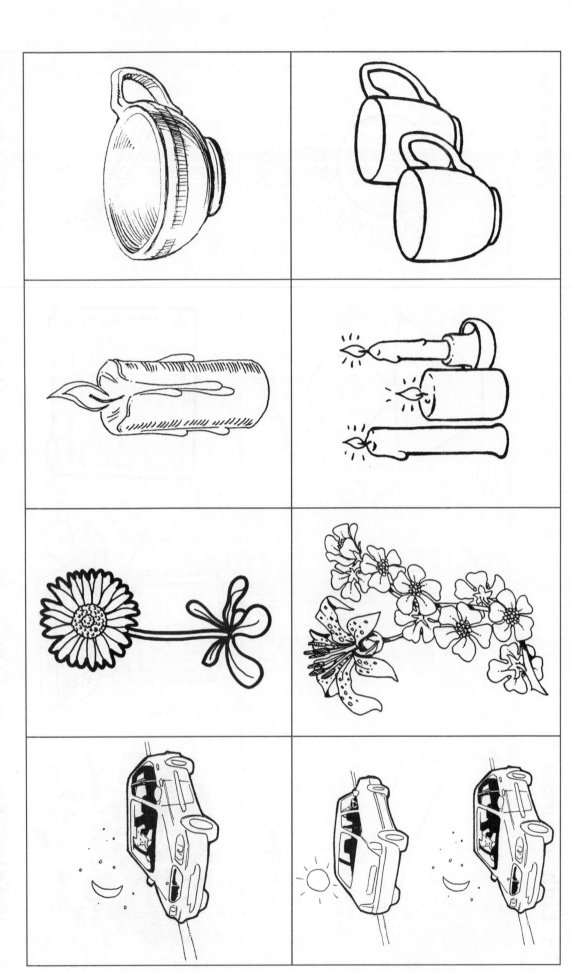

20 **Boy and girl**

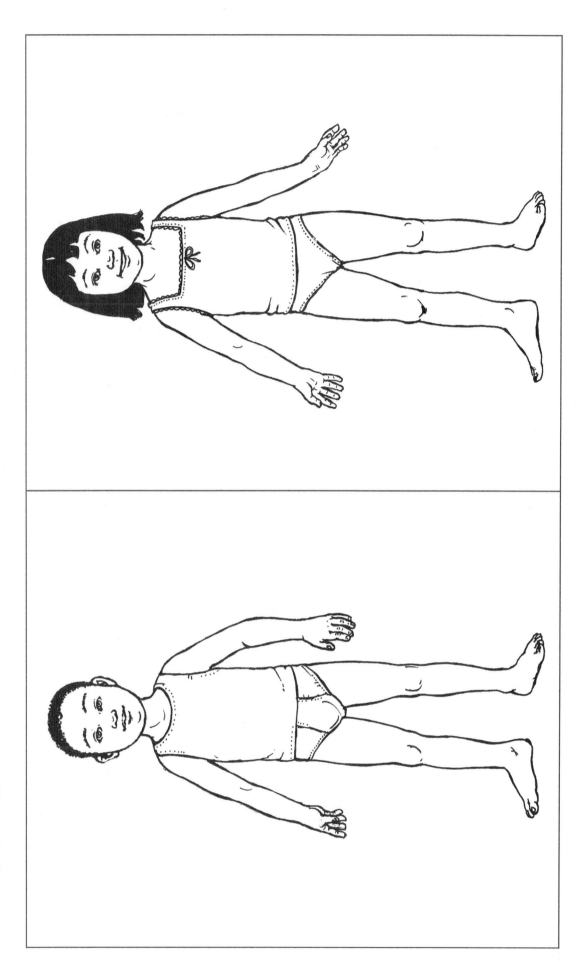

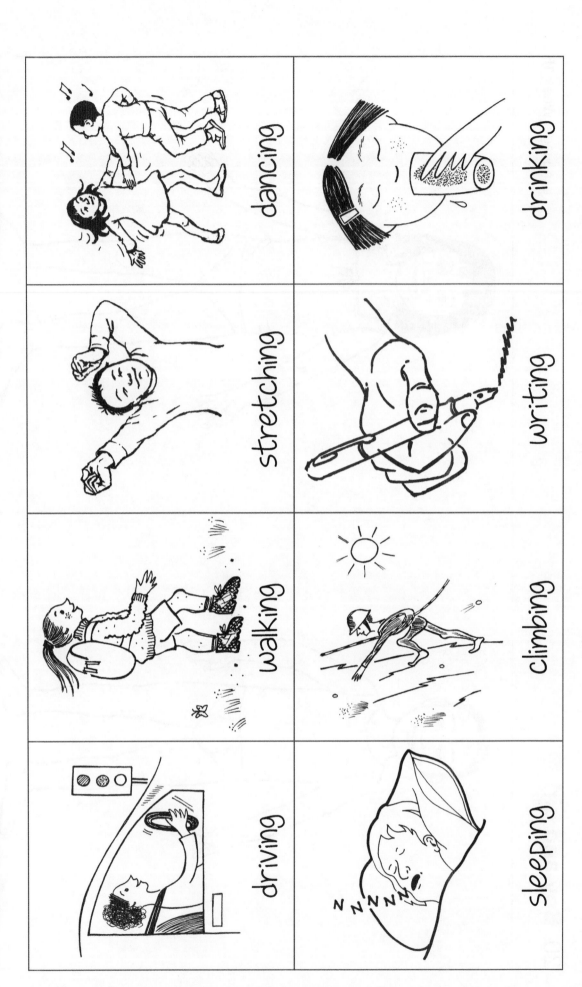

Language **Weeks 16, 17, 20**

dancing

drinking

stretching

writing

walking

climbing

driving

sleeping

21 **Actions (2)**

Language **Week 17**

Colour in the fruit.

22 **Fruit**

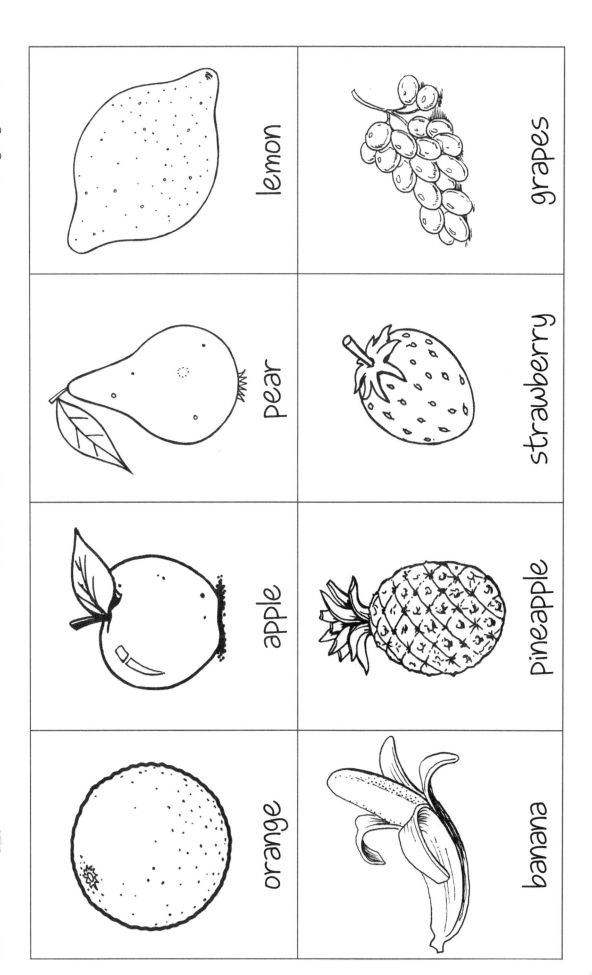

lemon

grapes

pear

strawberry

apple

pineapple

orange

banana

23 **Missing parts**

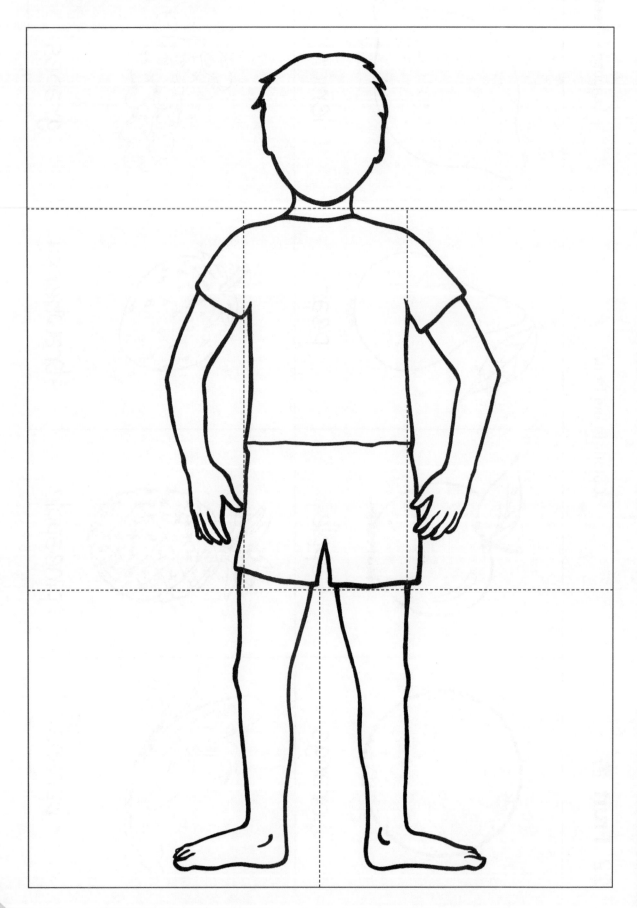

Language **Weeks 17 and 19**

Colour in the vegetables.

24 **Vegetables**

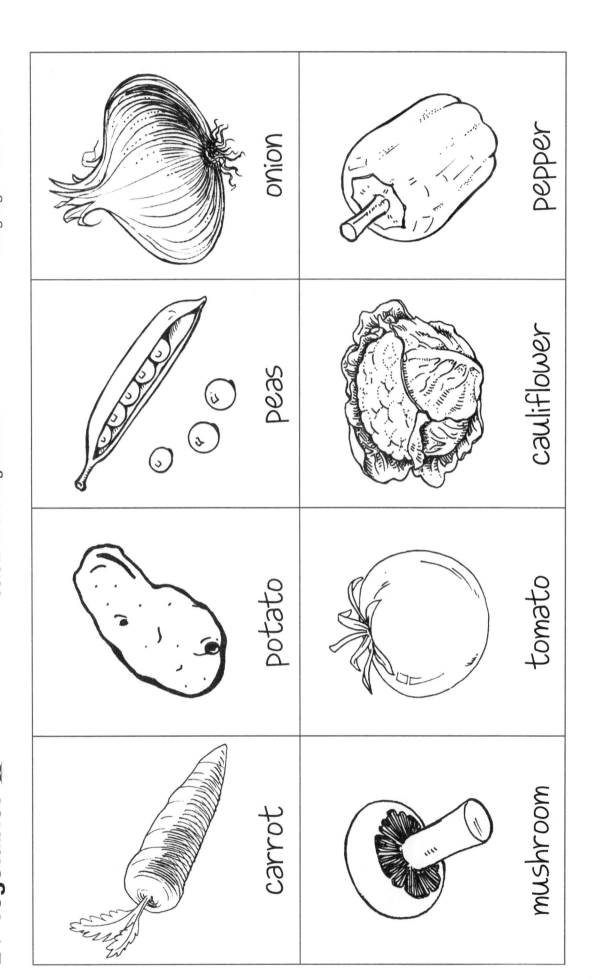

onion

pepper

peas

cauliflower

potato

tomato

carrot

mushroom

Language **Weeks 7, 19, 22**

25 **Lotto board (2)**

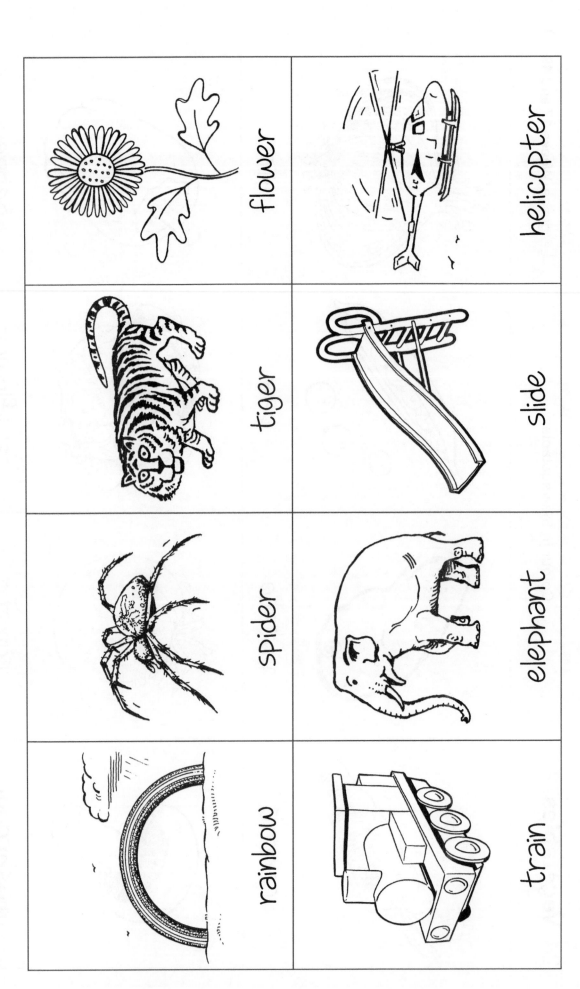

flower

helicopter

tiger

slide

spider

elephant

rainbow

train

26 **Tools**

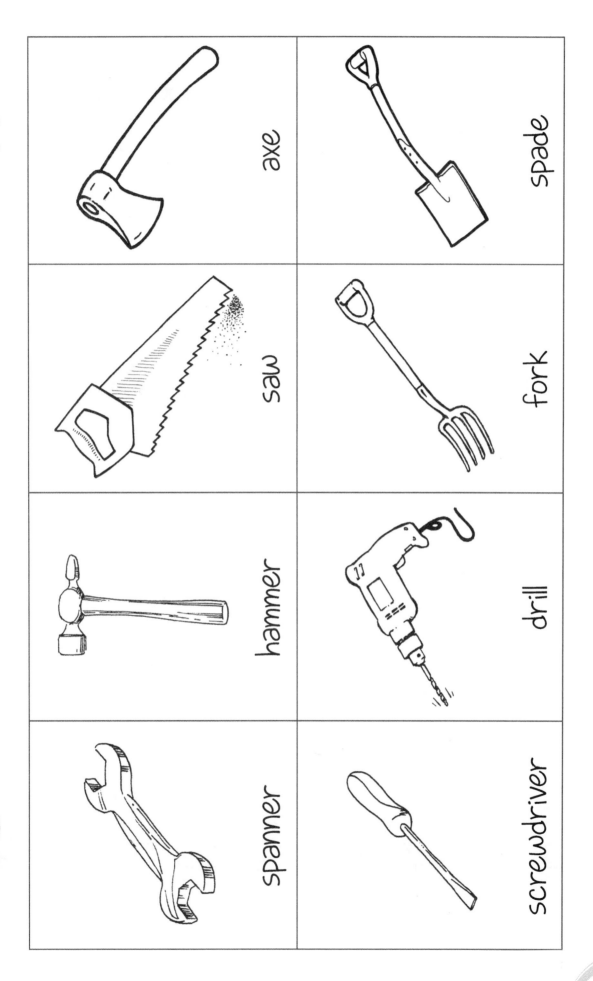

axe

spade

saw

fork

hammer

drill

spanner

screwdriver

Language **Week 20**

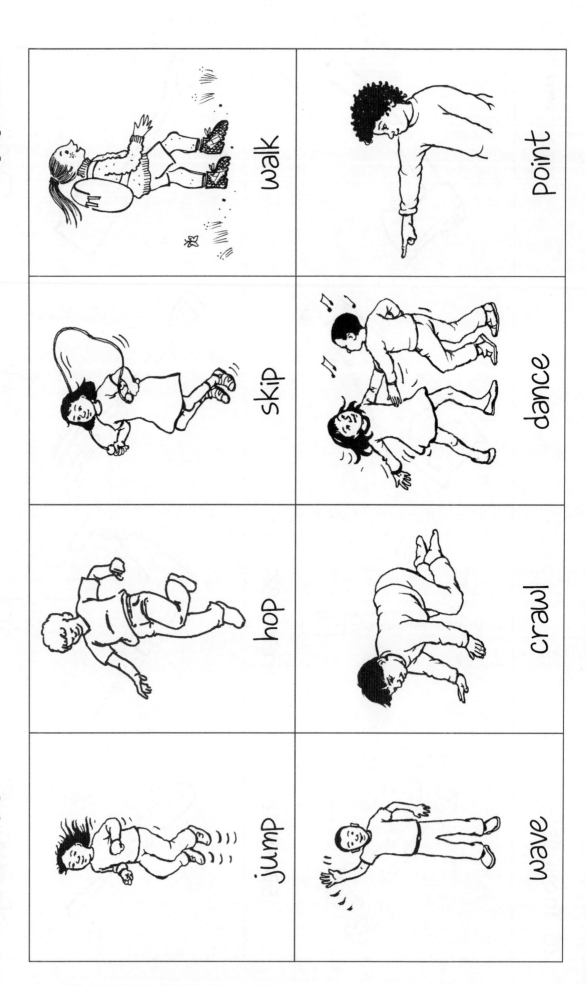

walk

point

skip

dance

hop

crawl

jump

wave

27 **Actions (3)**

Language **Weeks 21 and 24**

28 **Baby animals**

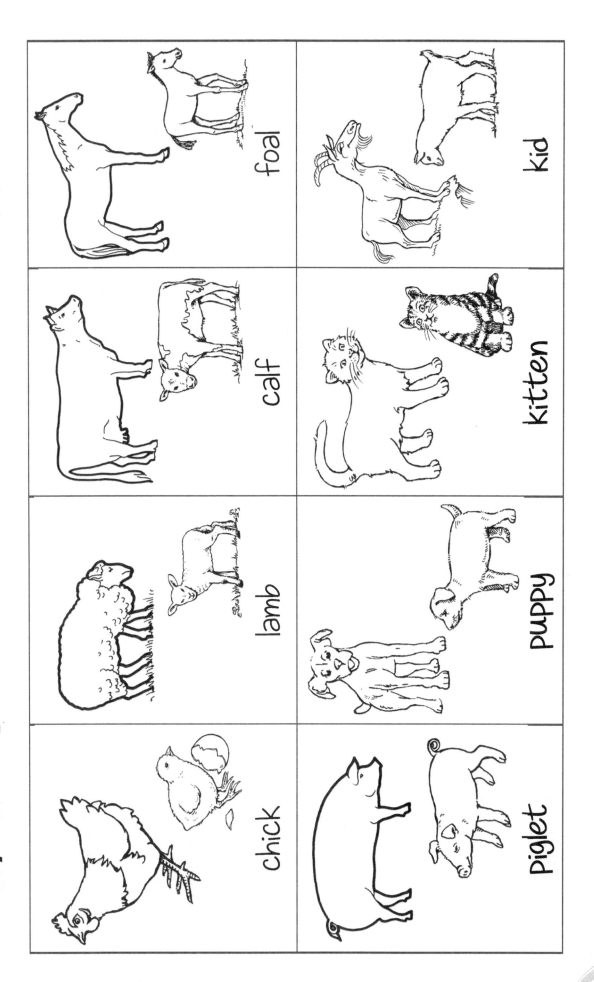

foal

kid

calf

kitten

lamb

puppy

chick

piglet

Language **Week 22**

29 **Shapes**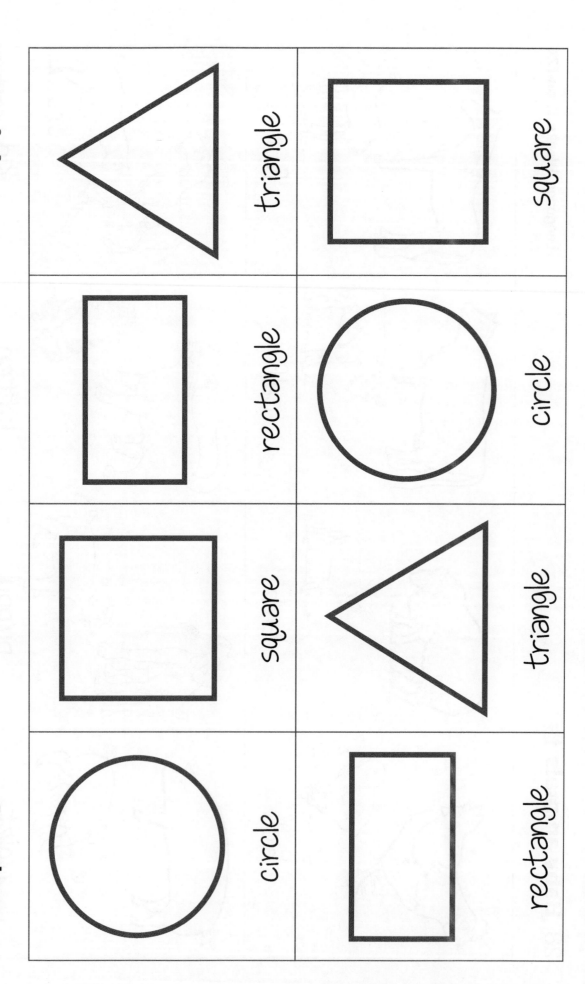

triangle

square

rectangle

circle

square

triangle

circle

rectangle

Language **Week 22**

30 **Lotto board (3)**

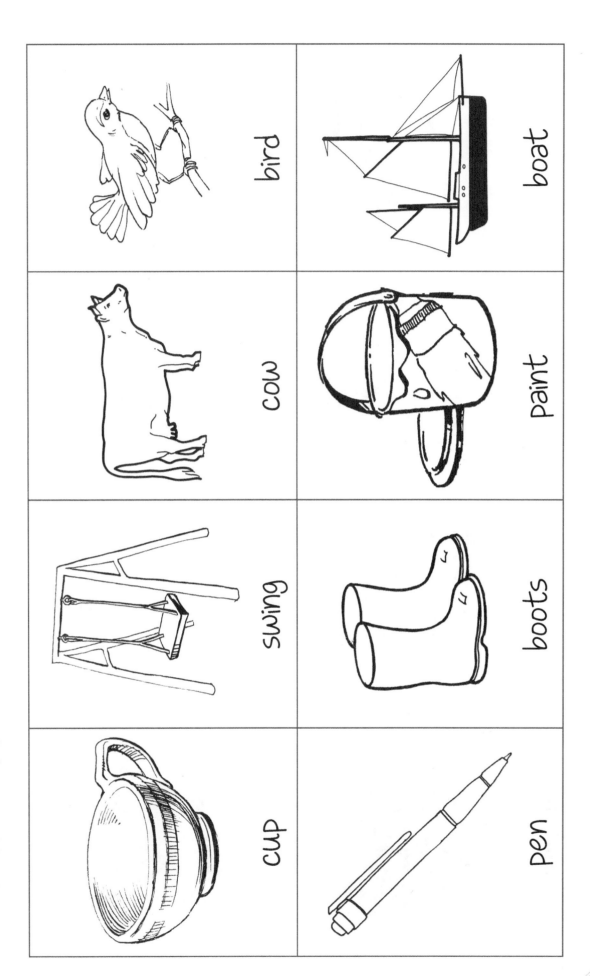

bird

boat

cow

paint

swing

boots

cup

pen

31 **Animals (2)**

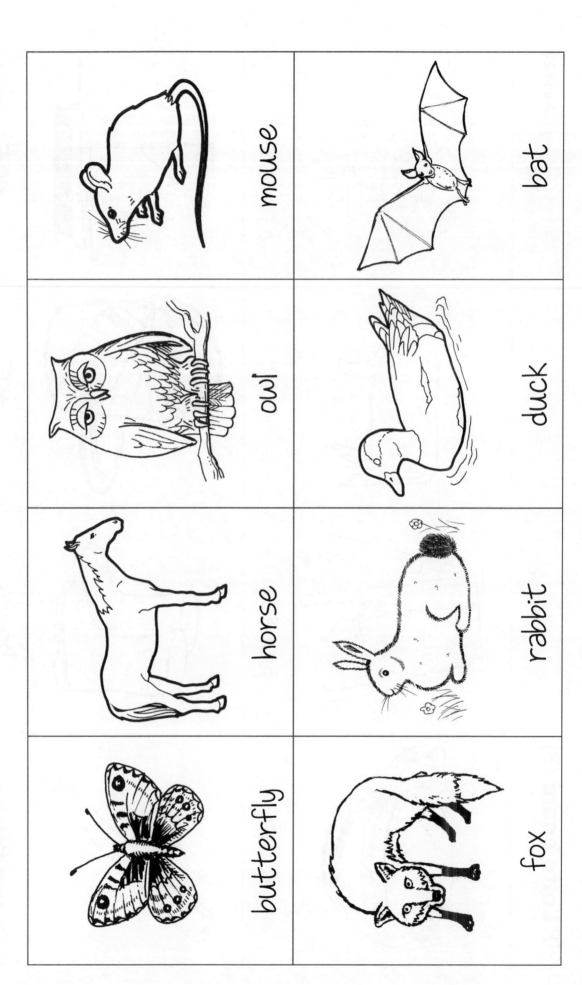

mouse

bat

owl

duck

horse

rabbit

butterfly

fox

32 **The farm**

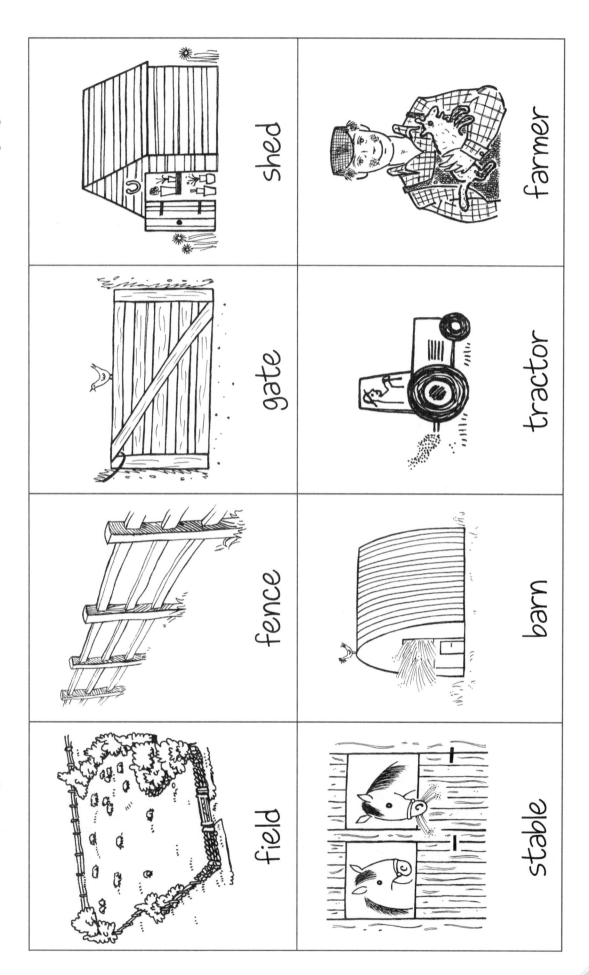

shed

farmer

gate

tractor

fence

barn

field

stable

Routledge
Taylor & Francis Group

Language **Week 25**

33 **Category cards (1)**

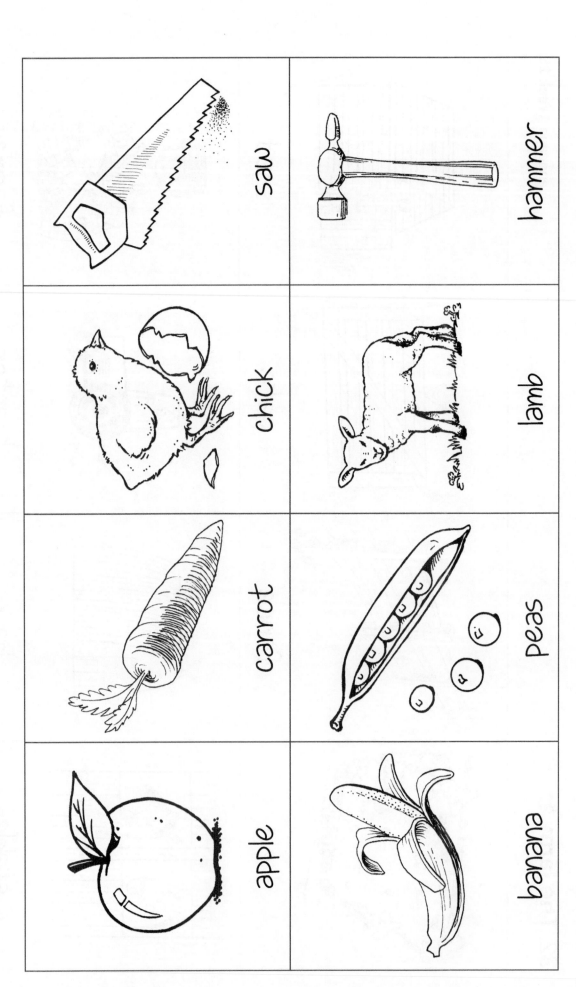

saw

hammer

chick

lamb

carrot

peas

apple

banana

34 Parts of a tree

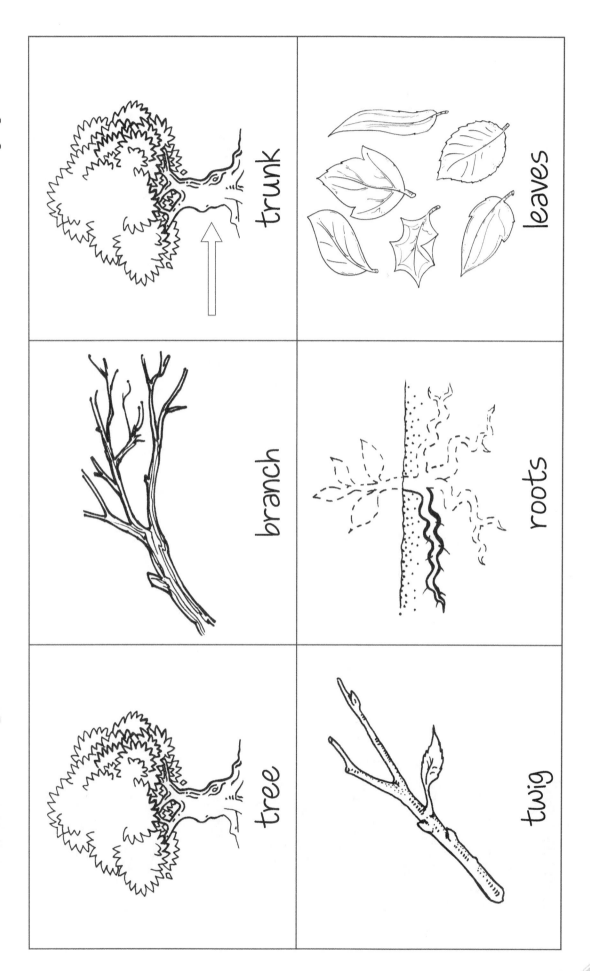

trunk

leaves

branch

roots

tree

twig

Language **Weeks 26 and 27**

35 **Happy/sad cards**

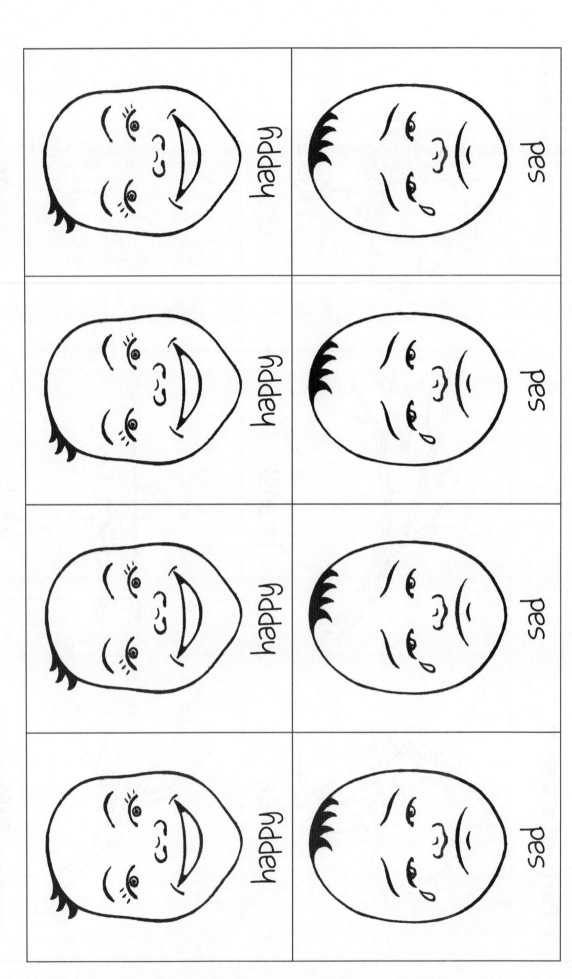

36 **Parts of a plant**

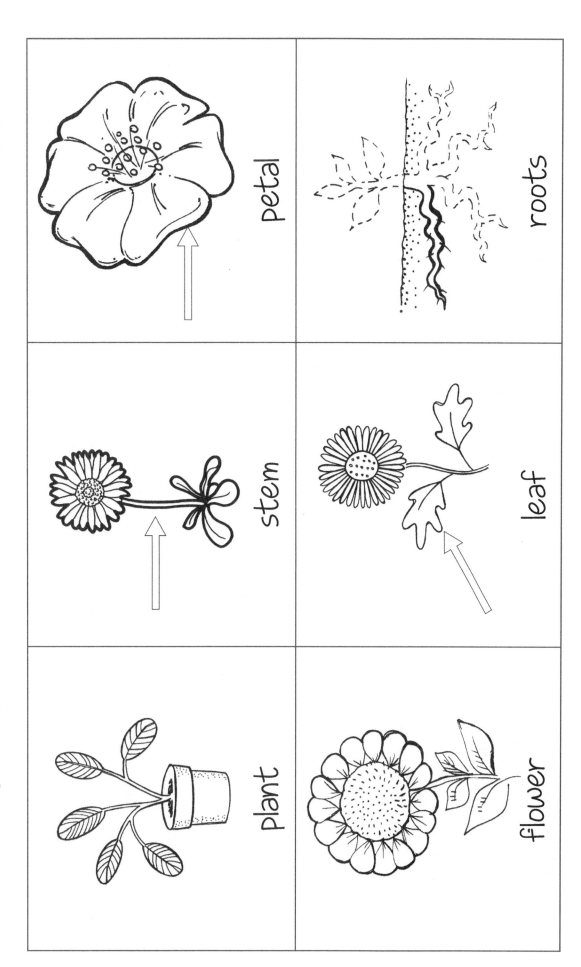

petal

roots

stem

leaf

plant

flower

37 **Description clues**

orange — It is round, juicy and is a fruit.

elephant — It is an animal. It is big, it has a trunk.

tree — It grows, it has branches, you can climb it.

aeroplane — It can fly. It can take you on holiday, it has wings.

cat — It is an animal, it is small. It has whiskers, it goes 'miaow'.

book — It is made of paper and stiff card. You can open it, you can read it.

door — It is made of wood. You can open and close it, you open it to get into your house.

coat — You wear it. It keeps you warm outdoors, it fastens with buttons or a zip.

flower — It smells nice, it grows in the garden, it is colourful.

spoon — You find it in the kitchen. It is made of metal, you use it to eat soup.

Language **Week 28**

38 **Seaside**

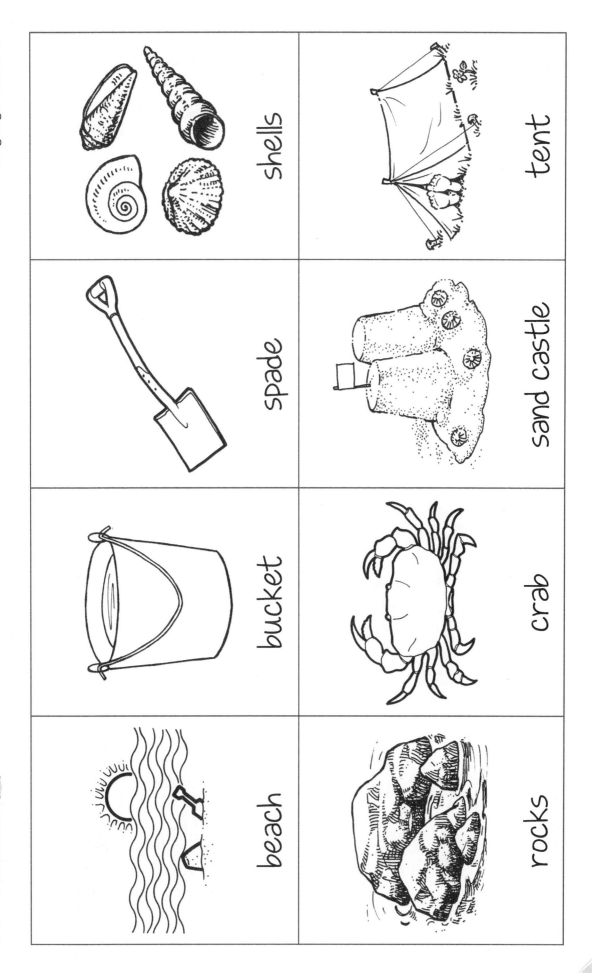

shells

tent

spade

sand castle

bucket

crab

beach

rocks

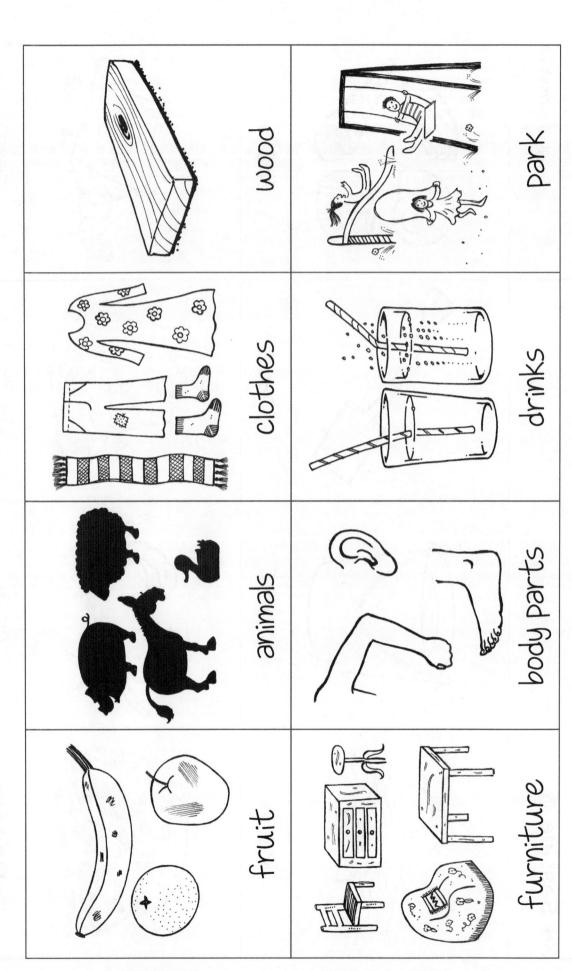

Language **Week 28**

39 **Category cards (2)**

wood

park

clothes

drinks

animals

body parts

fruit

furniture

Language **Week 28**

40 Picture pairs (1)

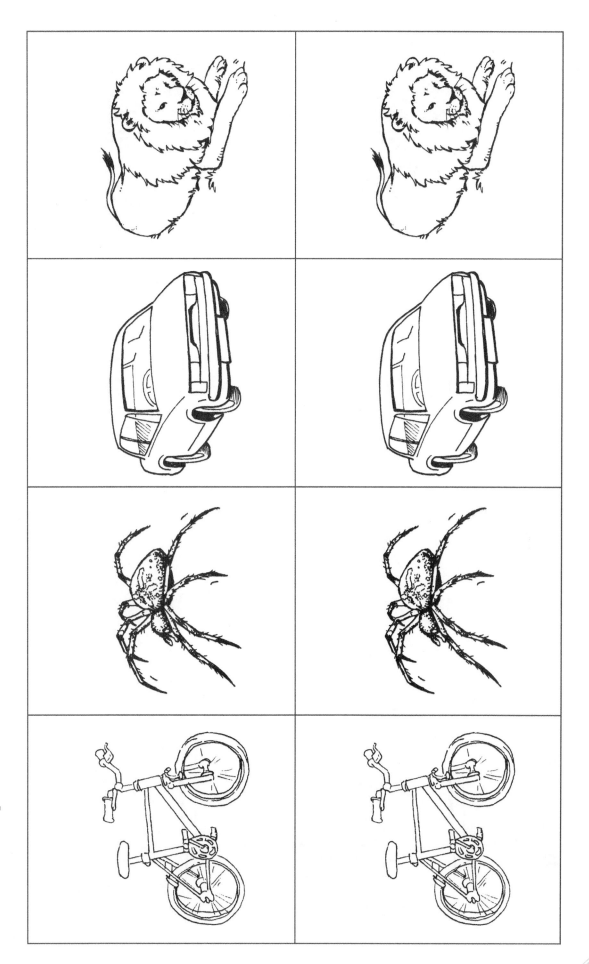

Language **Week 28**

41 **Picture pairs (2)**

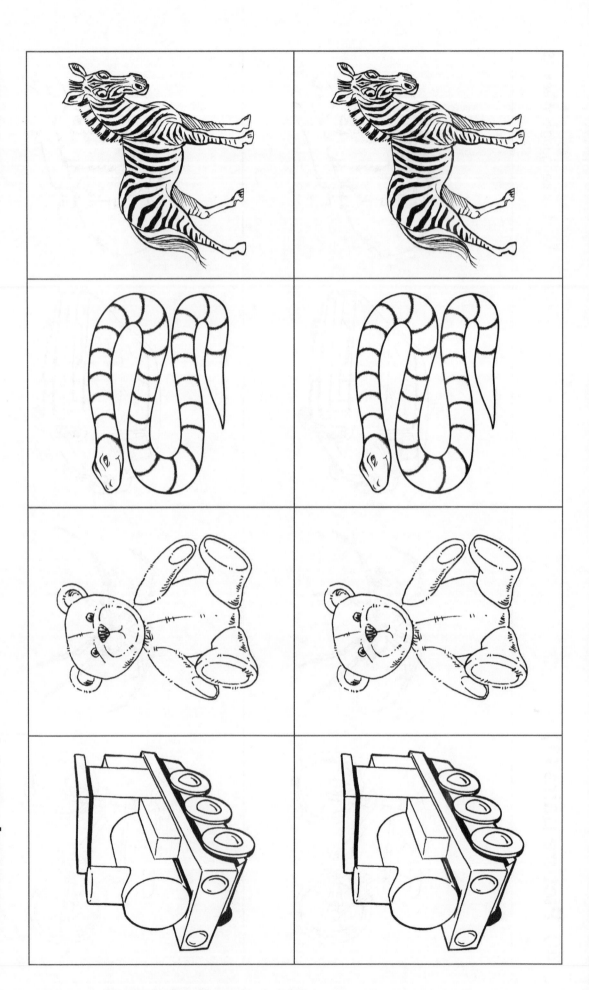

Language **Week 29**

42 **Clothes for a hot day**

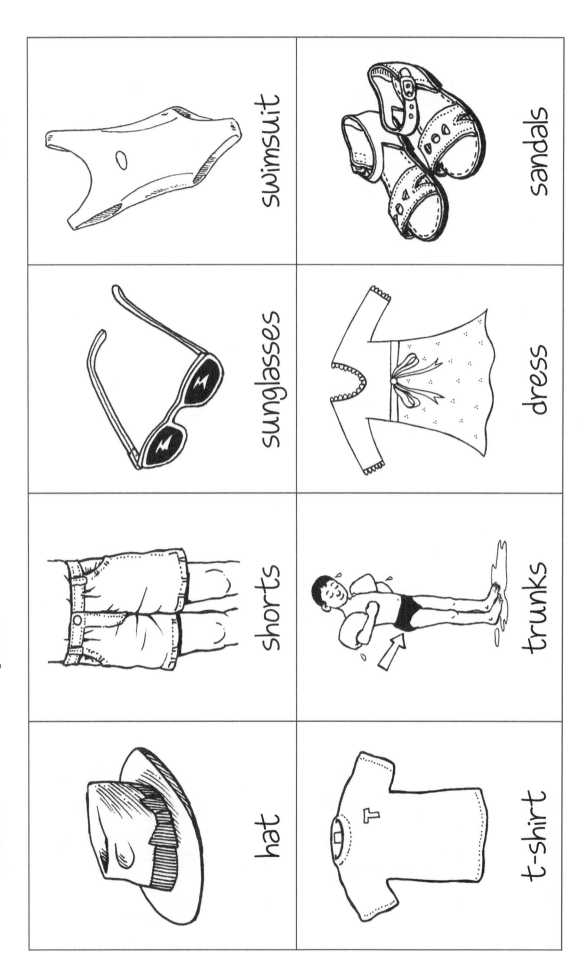

swimsuit

sandals

sunglasses

dress

shorts

trunks

hat

t-shirt

Routledge
Taylor & Francis Group

Language **Week 29**

43 **Clothes for a cold day** 🏠

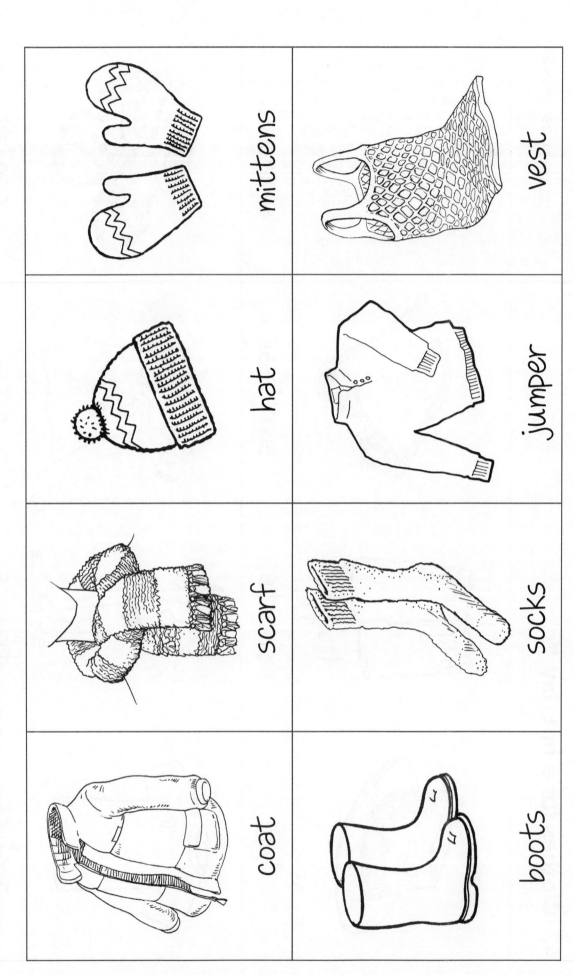

mittens

vest

hat

jumper

scarf

socks

coat

boots

Language **Week 30**

44 **Parts of your body**

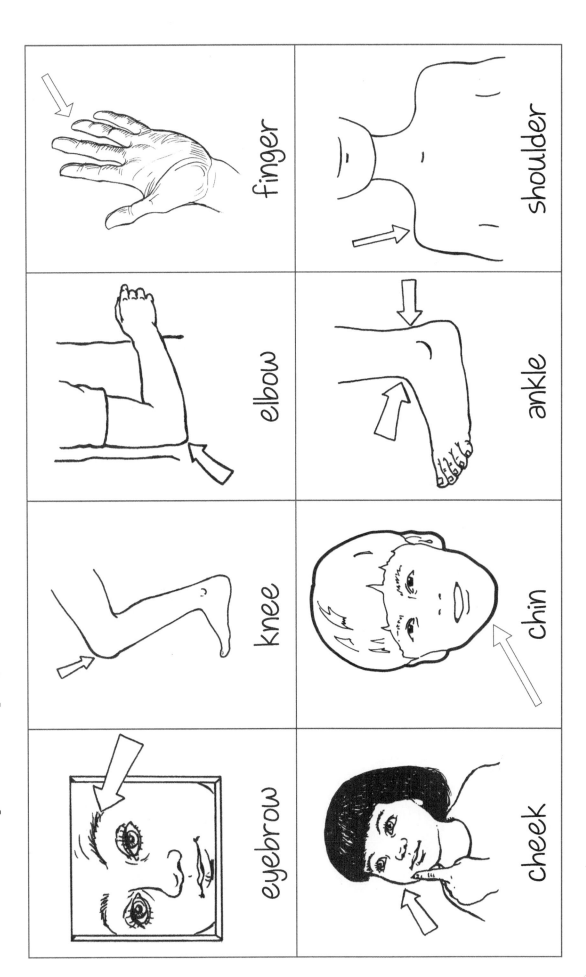

finger

shoulder

elbow

ankle

knee

chin

eyebrow

cheek

Sound Awareness Templates
45–70

Sound Awareness **Weeks 7 and 8**

45 **Yes/no or happy/sad faces**

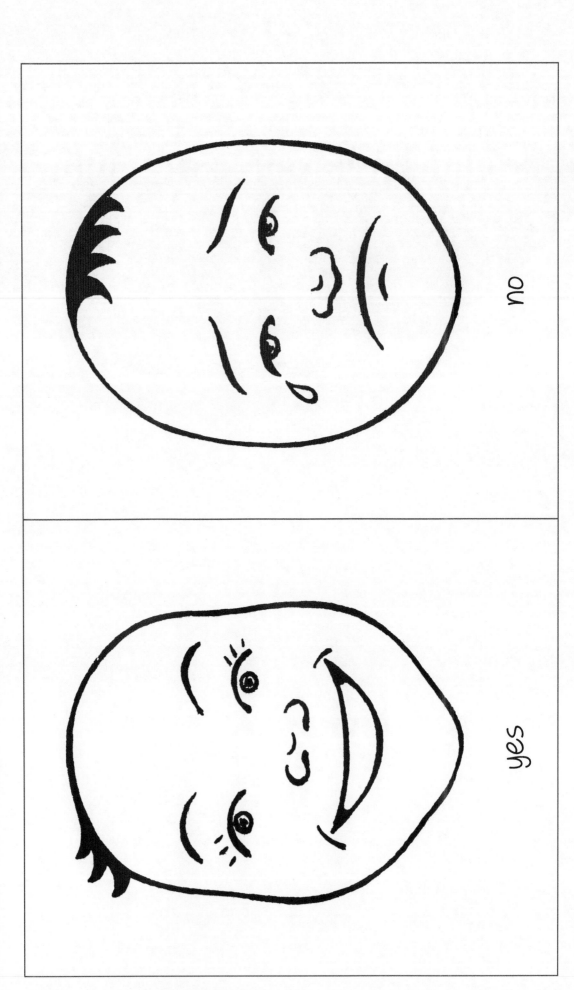

no

yes

46 **Rhyme sheet**   Sound Awareness **Weeks 9 and 10**

List 1

Target word	Which one rhymes?	
go	toe	cup
two	cat	boo
pear	bear	tap
book	ring	look
tap	cap	shoe
door	fox	more
boat	coat	bag
fish	pot	dish
bee	pea	soap
ten	soup	pen
pie	buy	four
man	sheep	van

List 2

Target word	Which one rhymes?		
fish	car	dish	train
book	kite	cook	dish
key	sea	pen	lid
hen	pot	bed	ten
gate	car	date	bag
show	mow	duck	cup
pen	book	spoon	den
glue	tree	blue	bin
far	bar	door	train
goat	cake	top	coat

Sound Awareness **Week 11**

47 **Lotto board (4)**

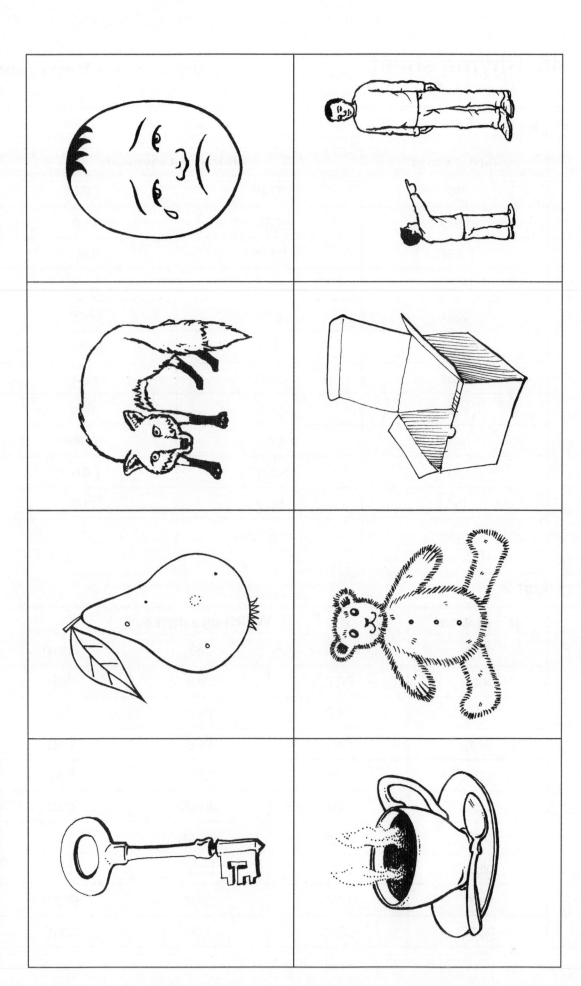

48 **Rhyme and riddle completion**

1 Rhyme completion sentences (Week 11)

I sit on a log, I am a d....	Mum likes to bake a yummy c....
Knock four, on the d....	Sit on the wall and hold the b....
I am a cat, I sit on the m....	I like to see the stripy b....
I found my bear next to my p....	I opened the box and saw a f....
In my den, I have a magic p....	I went to the shop and the balloon went p....
My name's Joe, I have a little t....	I like to stick with glue, my favourite colour is bl....

2 Rhyme riddles (Week 12)

It rhymes with spoon, at night you see the	It rhymes with bun, in the sky is the yellow ....
It rhymes with toes, you smell with your	It rhymes with door, I'm the number ....
It rhymes with cook, I like to read a	It rhymes with key, I like to drink ....
I can go far, when I drive my	It rhymes with boat, it's time to get my ....

49 **Word lists**

1 One-syllable words

car
spade
shoe
bird
train
dog
duck
bag

2 Two-syllable words

teddy
finger
flower
apple
toilet
milkshake
bucket
digger

3 Two one-syllable words together (Week 12 only)

blue car
big cup
more juice
go home
no sweets
my doll
your cup
red boat

Sound Awareness **Week 12**

50 **Lotto board (5)**

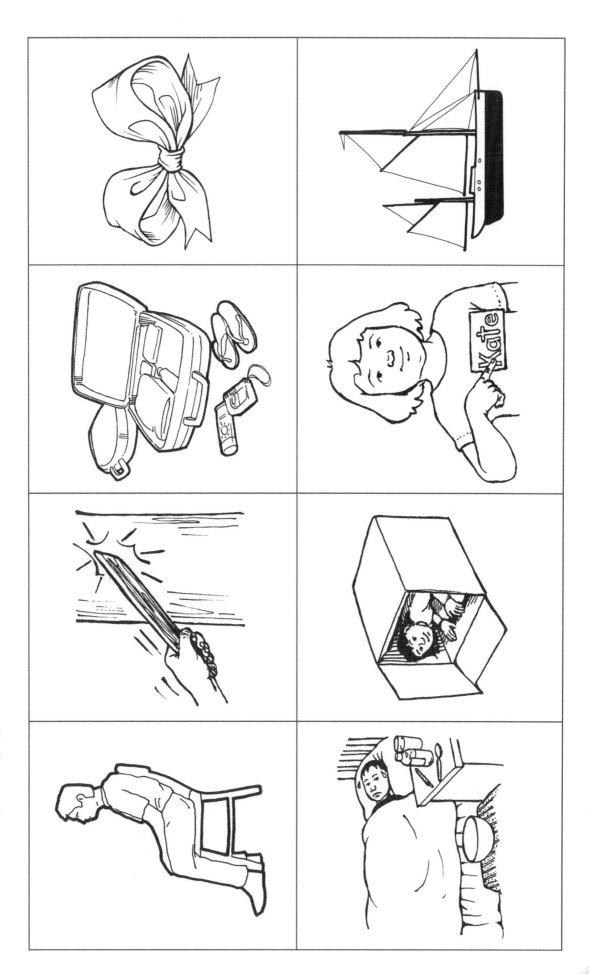

Routledge
Taylor & Francis Group

Sound Awareness **Weeks 13 and 14**

51 **Rhyme pictures (1)**

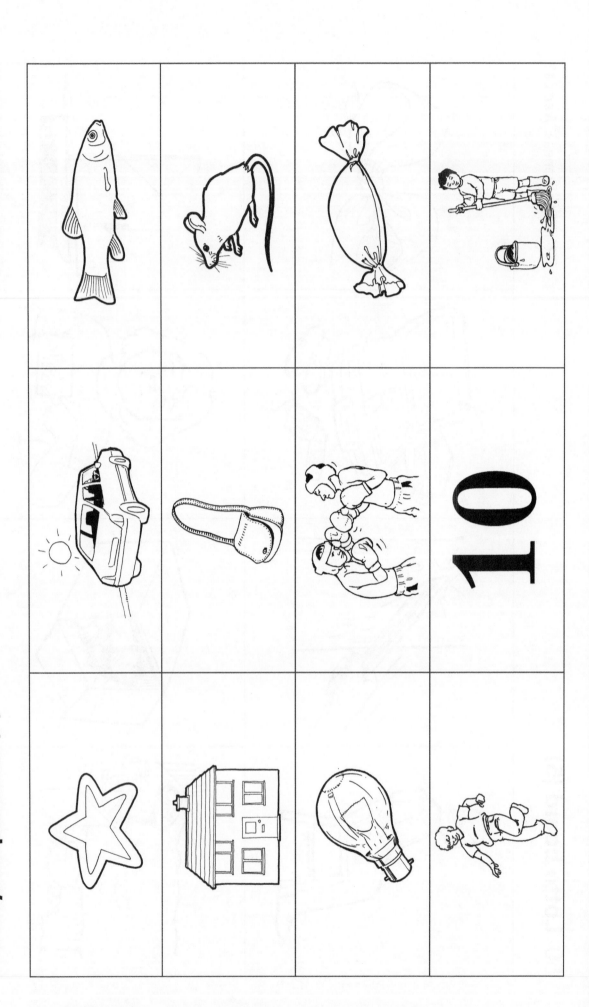

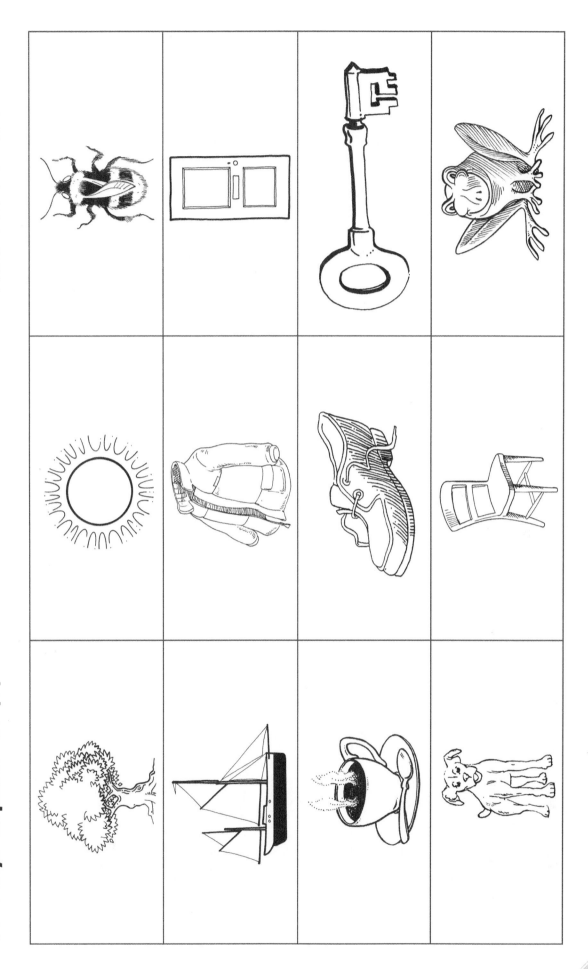

Sound Awareness **Weeks 13 and 14**

52 **Rhyme pictures (2)**

53 Lists of words and phrases

Sound Awareness **Weeks 13, 14, 15, 16, 17, 18**

1 Two-word phrases: one- and two-syllable words (Week 13)

mummy works	red jumper	more bubbles	no biscuits	small flower	daddy drives	little boat	my apple	

2 Three-word phrases: one-syllable words (Week 14)

dad is big	the blue train	go to school	get the cup	more juice please	in my house	on the chair	no more sweets	

3 Three separate words (Weeks 15, 16, 17)

car	duck	pen
tree	sock	book
train	bell	jumper
door	blue	stop
sweet	mouse	ladder
monkey	slide	clown
man	fox	table
apple	shoe	clock
cow	table	phone

4 Three-word phrases: mixed number of syllables (Weeks 15 and 18)

it is raining	go home now	my teddy jumps	no more juice	get that ball	here is dad	are you happy?	you are running	

54 **Cat story**

There was once a black **cat** who loved his milk in the morning.

The little girl came down the stairs and saw the **cat** in the kitchen.

'Hello **cat**!' she said, but the **cat** did not move.

The little girl stroked the **cat**. 'What's wrong?' she asked.

But the **cat** just sat there.

She found his ball but the **cat** still did not move.

Then she found his bell but the **cat** still did not move.

Then Mum came down the stairs and the **cat** followed her all the way to the fridge.

The **cat** miaowed loudly and Mum poured some milk into the **cat's** bowl.

The **cat** licked his mouth and drank all of the milk.

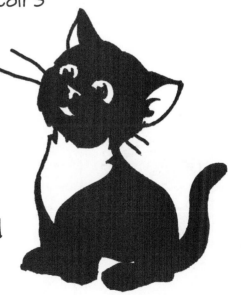

Sound Awareness **Week 15**

55 **Rhyme pictures (3)**

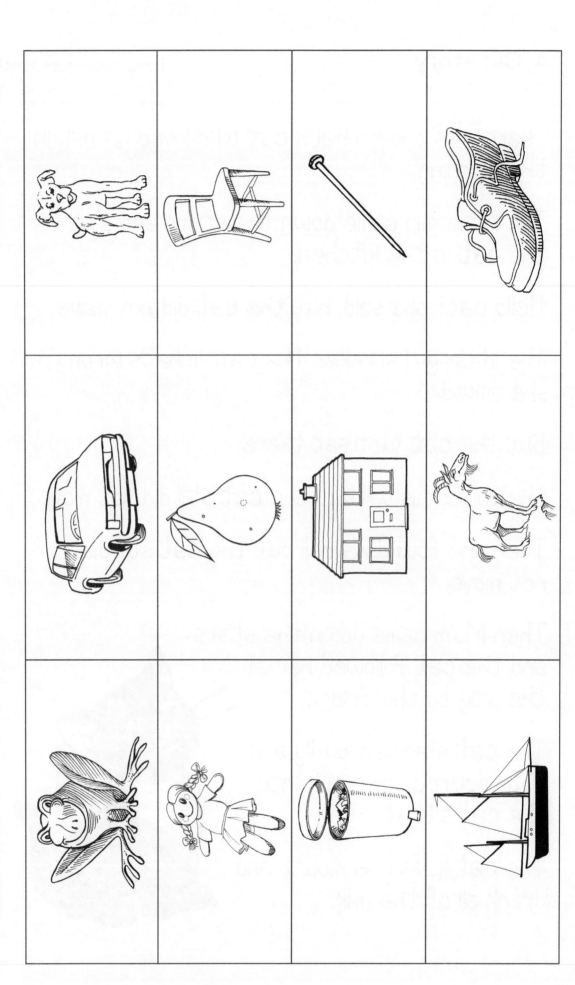

Sound Awareness **Week 15**

56 **Rhyme pictures (4)**

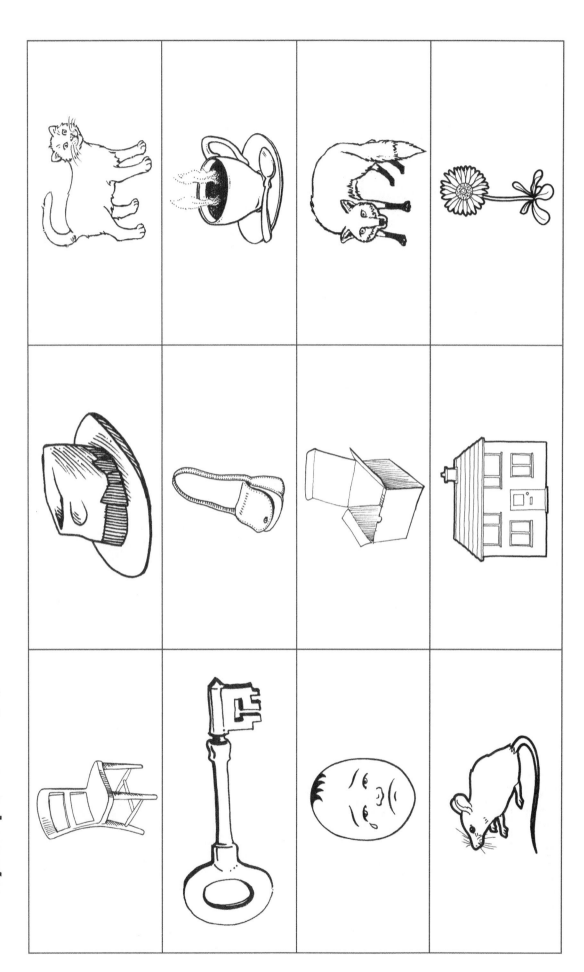

Sound Awareness **Weeks 16 and 17**

57 **Rhyming picture pairs (1)**

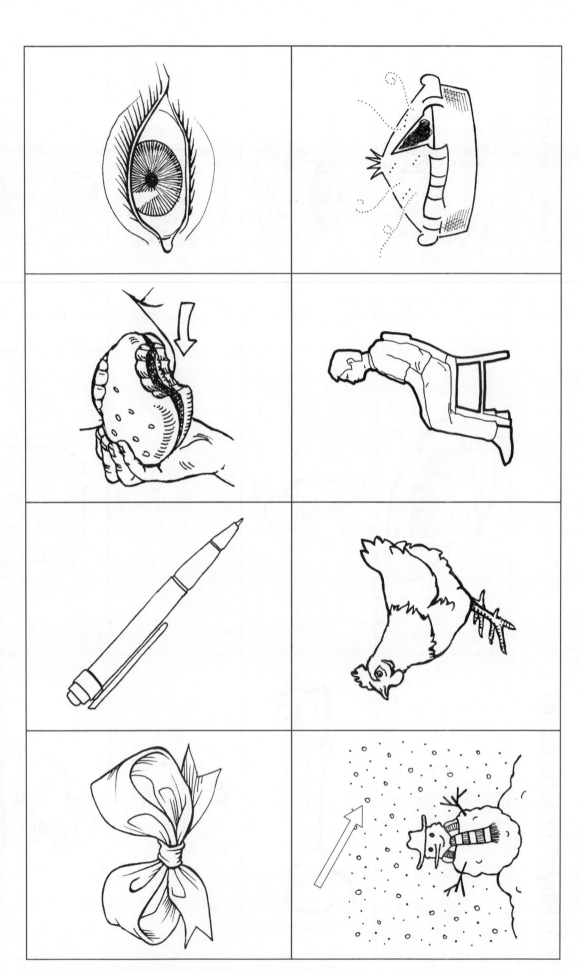

58 **Rhyming picture pairs (2)**

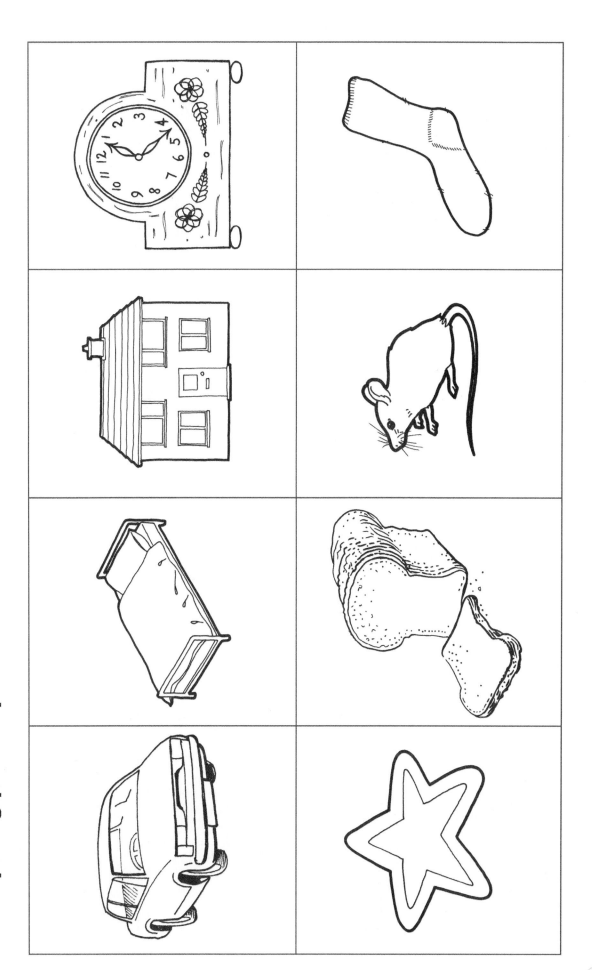

Routledge
Taylor & Francis Group

Sound Awareness **Weeks 15, 16, 17, 18, 27, 28, 29, 30**

59 **Train**

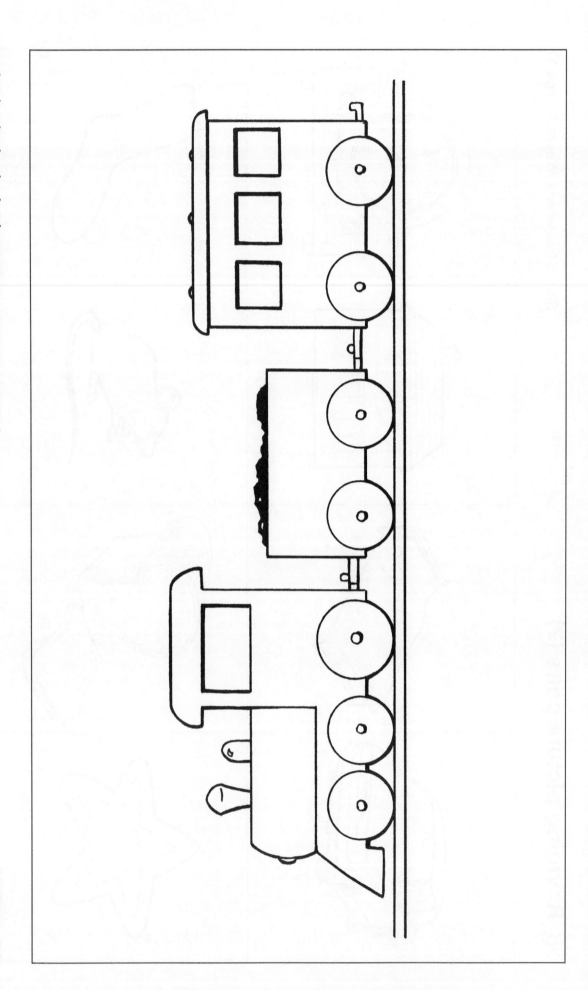

60 **Short sentences**

Sentence	Number of words
He jumped.	2
Help, please!	2
Get down now!	3
It is red.	3
Mum is holding on.	4
The man is walking.	4
No more sweets today.	4
Dad jumped up quickly.	4
The lady stopped to look.	5
He hopped onto the step.	5
The car is moving fast.	5
Please turn the light off.	5

61 **Robot**

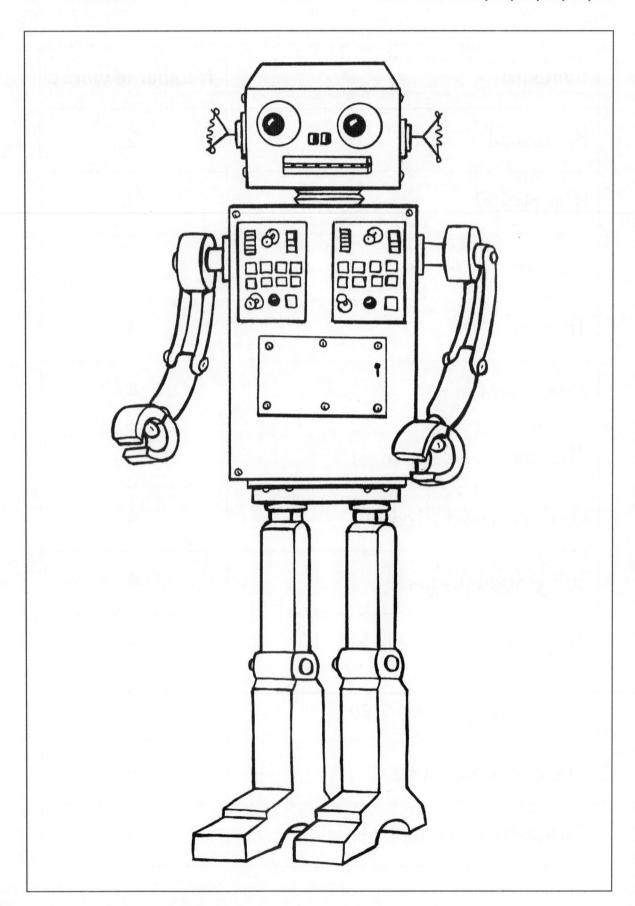

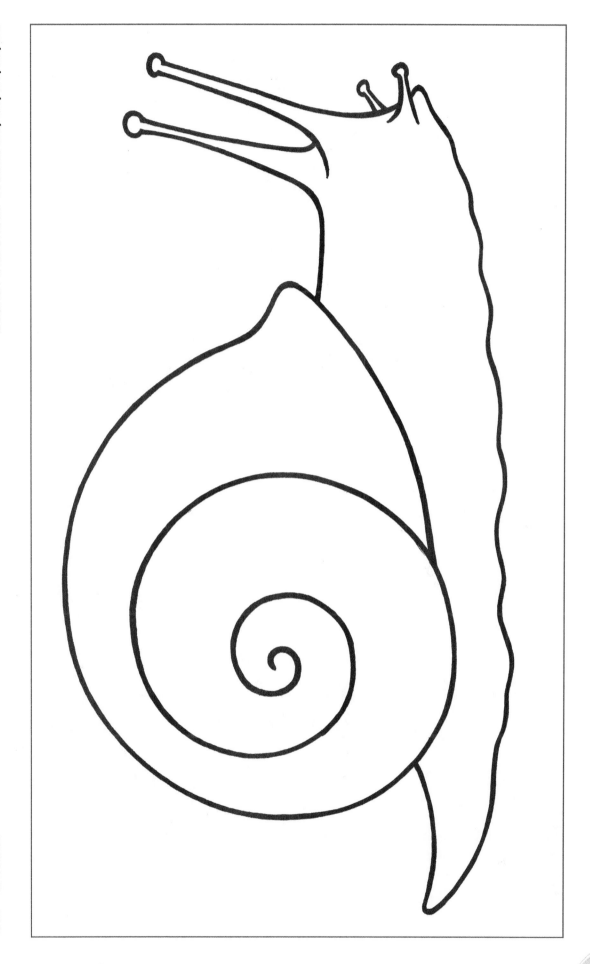

62 **Snail**

63 Two-syllable word pictures (1)

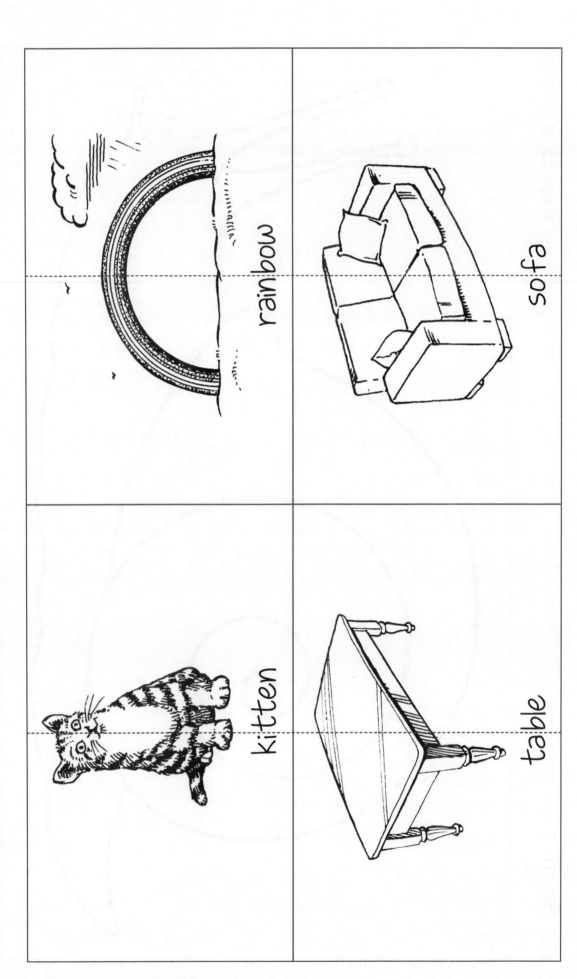

Sound Awareness **Week 22**

rainbow

sofa

kitten

table

64 Two-syllable word pictures (2)

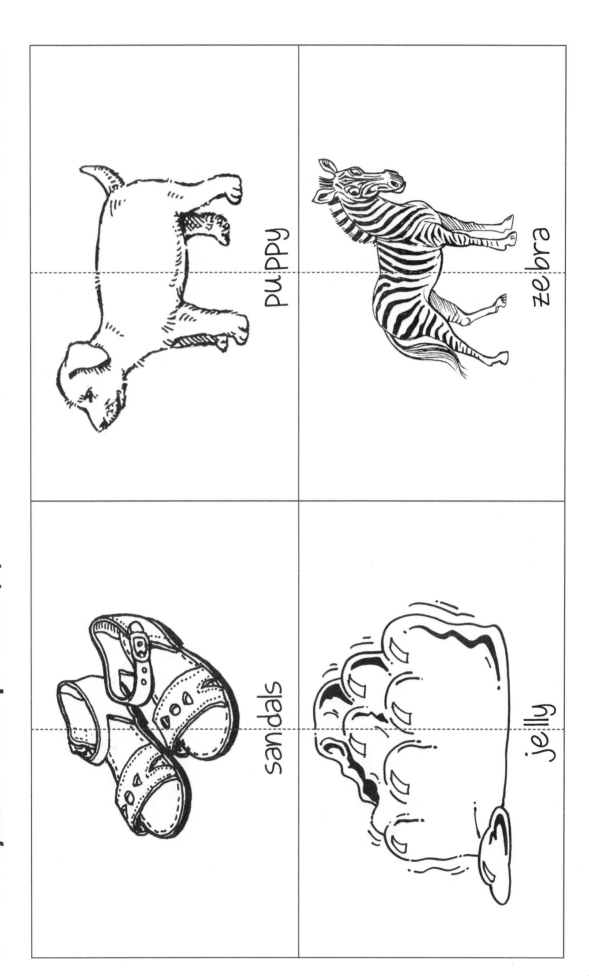

puppy

zebra

sandals

jelly

65 Three-syllable word pictures (1)

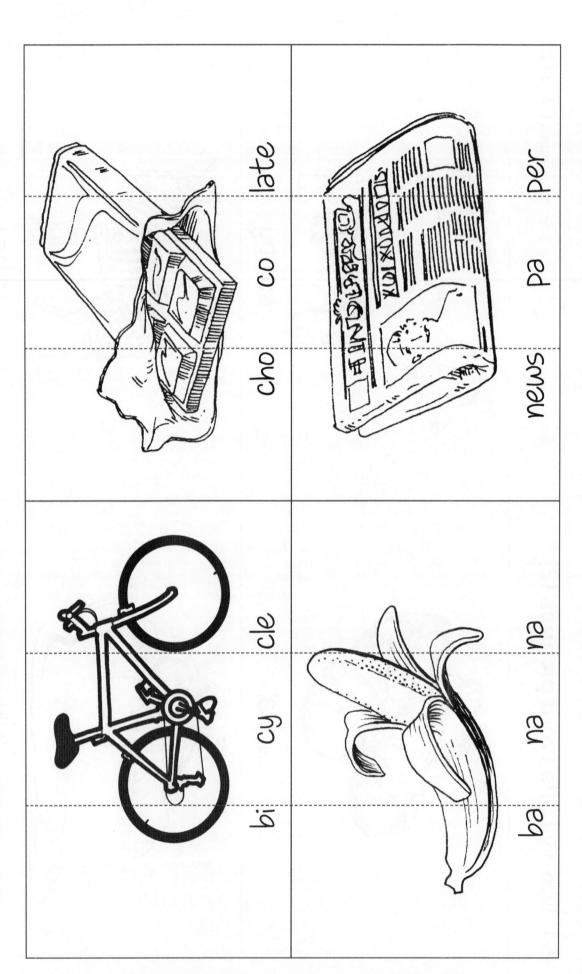

bi   cy   cle

ba   na   na

cho   co   late

news   pa   per

Sound Awareness **Week 23**

66 **Three-syllable word pictures (2)**

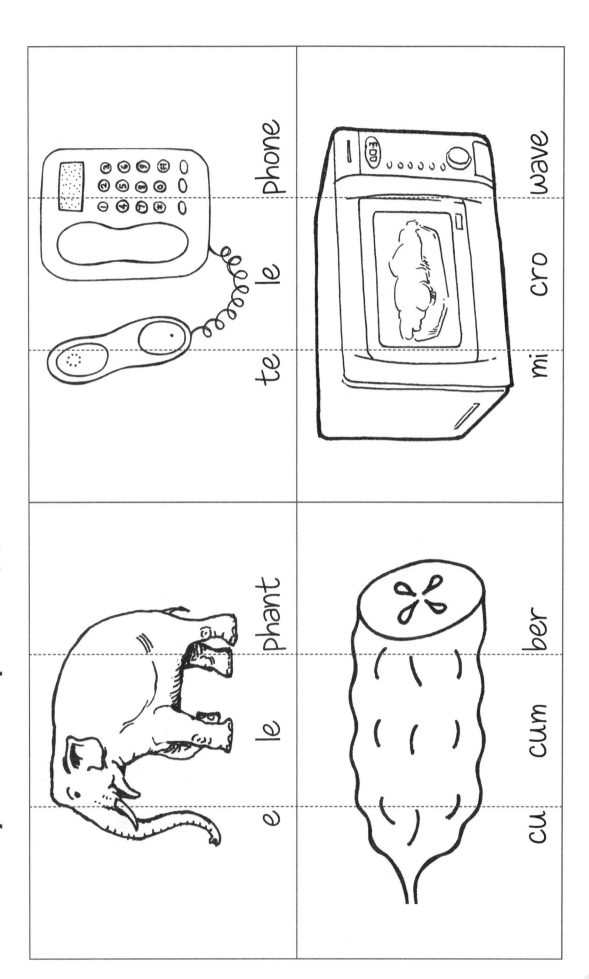

67 **Parrot**

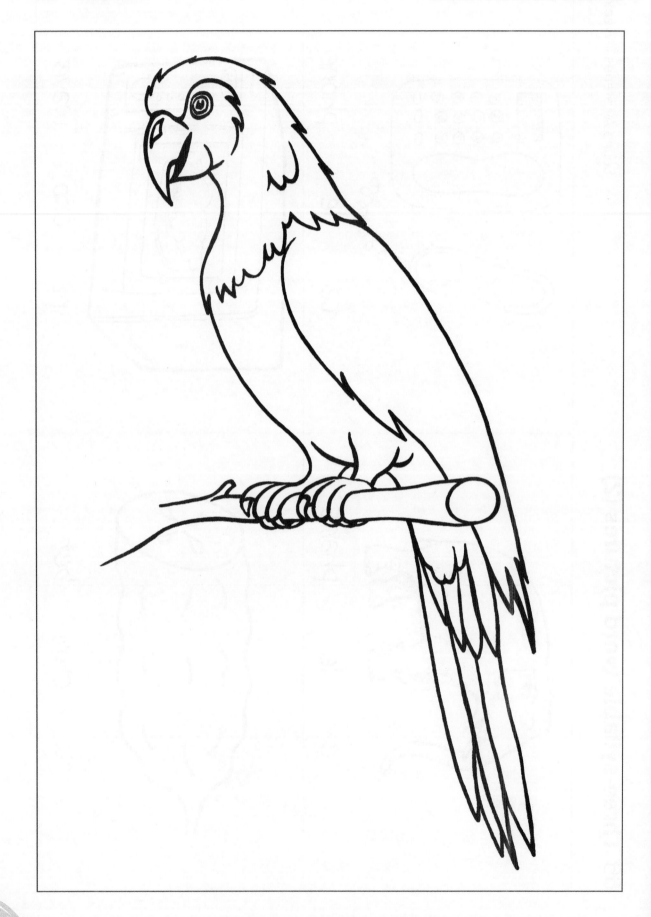

Sound Awareness **Weeks 25 and 26**

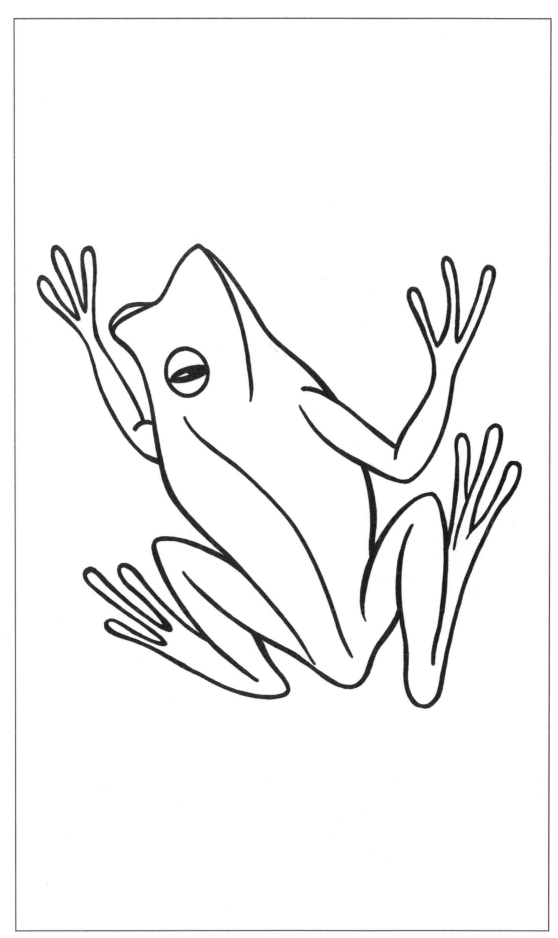

68 **Frog**

161

Sound Awareness **Week 27**

69 **Two-sound word pictures**

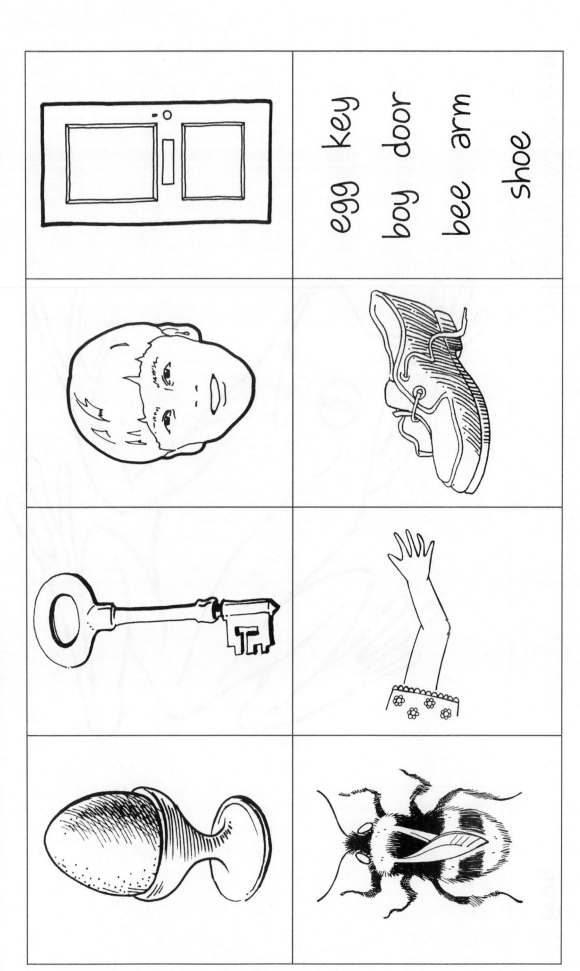

egg key

boy door

bee arm

shoe

Sound Awareness **Weks 28, 29, 30**

70 **Three-sound word pictures**

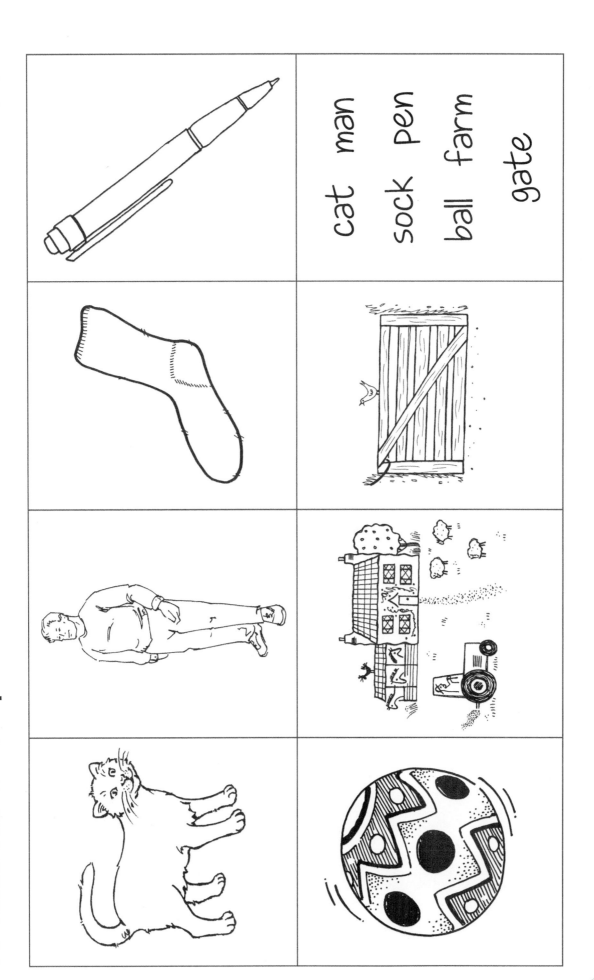

cat man
sock pen
ball farm
gate

Part 4

Programme Delivery Templates

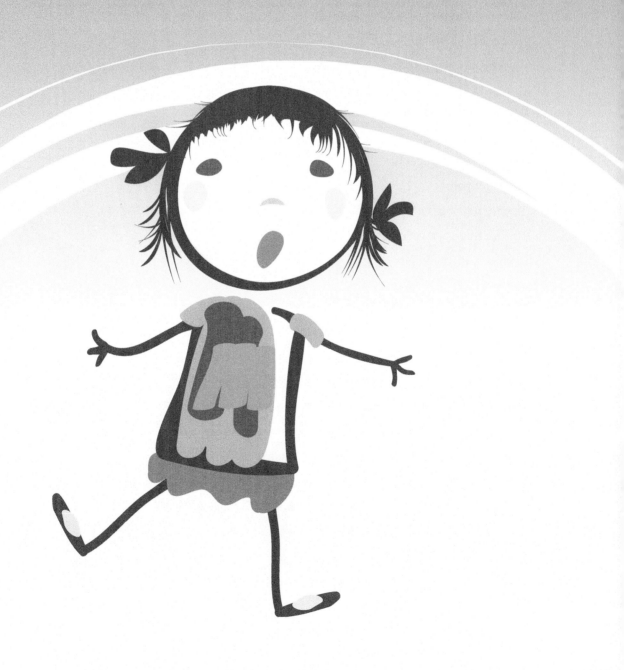

Contents

Record Sheets   **167**

Language Sessions Checklist   168

Sound Awareness Sessions Checklist   169

School Start Timetable   170

Child Evaluation Records   171

Starting the programme   **181**

Set-up meeting agenda   182

Training meeting agenda   184

Notes for parents   186

Tips for running the Language Sessions   187

Tips for running the Sound Awareness Sessions   188

Signs and symbols list   189

Handouts for home and class   **191**

Sample Service Agreement and Description   192

Handout for Home and Class: Language Sessions Weeks 1–6   196

Handout for Home and Class: Language Sessions Weeks 7–12   197

Handout for Home and Class: Language Sessions Weeks 13–18   198

Handout for Home and Class: Language Sessions Weeks 19–24   199

Handout for Home and Class: Language Sessions Weeks 25–30   200

Handout for Home and Class: Sound Awareness Sessions Weeks 1–6   201

Handout for Home and Class: Sound Awareness Sessions Weeks 7–12   202

Handout for Home and Class: Sound Awareness Sessions Weeks 13–18   203

Handout for Home and Class: Sound Awareness Sessions Weeks 19–24   204

Handout for Home and Class: Sound Awareness Sessions Weeks 25–30   205

Record Sheets

Language Sessions Checklist

Child's name: Date of birth:

School name: Class:

Completed by: Date of completion:

Decision:

Concepts	Rarely (0–40%)	Sometimes (41–80%)	Often (81% +)
A1 Knows big ☐ and little ☐			
A2 Names some colours			
A3 Knows ☐ more ☐ no more ☐ before ☐ after ☐ first ☐ last			
A4 Knows concepts of shapes ☐ ○ △			
A5 Knows ☐ many ☐ less ☐ bigger			
Vocabulary	**Rarely (0–40%)**	**Sometimes (41–80%)**	**Often (81% +)**
B1 Can name familiar items in class (eg pencil, scissors) and body parts (eg nose, mouth, legs)			
B2 Can follow verbal instructions containing actions, eg hop, climb, cut, skip, jump (no use of gesture by the adult)			
B3 Can sort objects into two groups according to category (relate to topic work, eg fruit/not fruit; wood/not wood)			
B4 Can give five words in a category, eg animals, food			
B5 Can give the meaning (function and features) of a topic word recently taught in class, eg What is a mini-beast?			
Total of items in column three 'often' = (A score of 4 or less indicates suitability for the group)			

The following factors may give additional reason for including the child in the Language Group: (circle as appropriate)

Attention	not a concern	a cause for concern
Following instructions	not a concern	a cause for concern
Social interaction	not a concern	a cause for concern

Sound Awareness Sessions Checklist

Child's name: _____ Date of birth: _____

School name: _____ Class: _____

Completed by: _____ Date of completion: _____

Decision: _____

Sound Awareness	Rarely (0–40%)	Sometimes (41–80%)	Often (81% +)
C1 Can walk three steps to show three words in a spoken sentence			
C2 Can clap out the syllables in own name			
C3 Can find two pictures of spoken words that rhyme			
C4 Can listen to spoken words and say if they do or do not rhyme			
C5 Can hear two sounds and blend to say the word (eg *e* + *gg* = egg)			
Speech	Rarely (0–40%)	Sometimes (41–80%)	Often (81% +)
C6 Speech can be clearly understood by unfamiliar adults			
Total of items in column three 'often' = (A score of 3 or less indicates suitability for the group)			

The following factors may give additional reason for including the child in the Sound Awareness Group: (circle as appropriate)

Attention not a concern a cause for concern

Following instructions not a concern a cause for concern

Social interaction not a concern a cause for concern

School Start Timetable

Date:

Staff

Title	Name	Contact details
Support staff, eg speech and language therapist (SLT)		
Reception class teacher		
Classroom assistant		
Classroom assistant		

Language group

Day of week	Time of day	Designated room

Children's names		
1	3	5
2	4	6

Sound Awareness group

Day of week	Time of day	Designated room

Children's names		
1	3	5
2	4	6

Child Evaluation Record

Language group

Learning objective Weeks 1–6	Evaluation Rarely/Sometimes/Often
To work as part of a group, taking turns and sharing	
To sustain attentive listening	
To follow rules in a group	
To match two pictures that are the same	
To investigate objects and materials using all of their senses	
To find the named item on request (toy animals or other toys, Christmas vocabulary, 'big'/'little')	
To extend word knowledge (understand and use the concept 'same' and the pronoun 'I', 'a' before an item and 'yes'/'no')	
Date:	**Child's name:**

Child Evaluation Record

Language group

Learning objective Weeks 7–12	Evaluation Rarely/Sometimes/Often
To be able to arrange items into categories	
To find named items on request (body parts and kitchenware)	
To find and name an item on request (clothes)	
To understand and use the concepts 'first', 'last' and 'different'	
To understand the prepositions 'on', 'in', 'under'	
To investigate objects and materials using touch	
To extend word knowledge, understand and use 'what', 'and', 'my', 'mine', 'your', 'you' and regular plural forms such as books/book	
Date:	Child's name:

Child Evaluation Record

Language group

Learning objective Weeks 13–18	Evaluation Rarely/Sometimes/Often
To find named item on request related to: (a) parts of a house (b) light	
To be able to understand and use the following concepts: (a) big, middle and little (for size) (b) bigger (c) prepositions 'behind' and 'in front of' (d) quick and slow	
To extend word knowledge of (understand and use): (a) 'he' and 'she' (b) regular plurals (c) 'his' and 'her' (d) 'and' with two verbs (e) 'no' with a noun	
To arrange items into categories according to the material that they are made from	
To ask questions using 'Who?' and 'Where?'	
Date:	Child's name:

Child Evaluation Record

Language group

Learning objective Weeks 19–24	Evaluation Rarely/Sometimes/Often
To arrange items into categories	
To understand the use of 'above'	
To extend word knowledge (asking 'What is it?' and 'Is it …?')	
To investigate objects and materials using touch (tools and shapes)	
To find a named item on request (in relation to tool vocabulary, shapes and animals)	
To understand the concepts of 'top', 'bottom', 'full', 'empty', 'push', 'pull' and 'below'	
To find two named items on request (related to baby animals)	
To extend word knowledge of 'him', 'her' and 'yours'; use of 'an' before a vowel; use of 'it is' for description	
To sustain attentive listening	
To name items (in relation to baby animals)	
Date:	**Child's name:**

Child Evaluation Record

Language group

Learning objective Weeks 25–30	Evaluation Rarely/Sometimes/Often
To find and name: (a) things at the farm (b) parts of a tree (c) parts of a plant (d) things at the seaside (e) clothes for a hot day	
To perform two actions in order	
To identify items within a given category	
To name an item: (a) in a given category (b) when given a description	
To extend word knowledge of: (a) 'happy' and 'sad' (b) 'many' (c) 'Who?'	
To remember two items after a short time delay	
To use the following in sentences: (a) 'Who?' (b) 'It is not' (c) 'here' (d) 'there' (e) 'or'	
To understand vocabulary related to body parts	
Date:	**Child's name:**

Child Evaluation Record

Sound Awareness group

Learning objective Weeks 1–6	Evaluation Rarely/Sometimes/Often
To listen for a word and respond appropriately	
To identify noises and sounds in the environment	
To join in with a familiar nursery rhyme	
To identify which musical instrument is played from a choice of two	
To understand the concept 'first'	
To understand the concept 'last'	
To be able to listen for a sound and respond appropriately	
To be aware of words that rhyme	
Date:	**Child's name:**

Child Evaluation Record

Sound Awareness group

Learning objective Weeks 7–12	Evaluation Rarely/Sometimes/Often
To listen for a sound from a choice of two and respond appropriately	
To identify which words rhyme	
To understand the concept 'last'	
To understand the concept 'middle'	
To be able to listen for a sound and respond appropriately	
To understand the concept and label for 'word'	
To give an example of a word that rhymes	
To move a counter for each word	
To correctly identify the named word from two that sound similar (eg bed/bread)	
Date:	**Child's name:**

Child Evaluation Record

Sound Awareness group

Learning objective Weeks 13–18	Evaluation Rarely/Sometimes/Often
To listen carefully to other people	
To identify which words rhyme	
To move a counter for each word	
To listen for a word in a story	
To give examples of words that rhyme	
To identify the first, middle and last words from a list of three	
To identify the first, last and middle words from a phrase	
Date:	Child's name:

Child Evaluation Record

Sound Awareness group

Learning objective Weeks 19–24	Evaluation Rarely/Sometimes/Often
To identify familiar sounds	
To give examples of words that rhyme	
To move a counter for each word spoken	
To listen for a word and respond appropriately	
To identify and say the separate syllables that make up words	
To listen for a sound and respond appropriately	
To listen to and follow an instruction	
To listen for a sound in a word and respond appropriately	
Date:	**Child's name:**

Child Evaluation Record

Sound Awareness group

Learning objective Weeks 25–30	Evaluation Rarely/Sometimes/Often
To listen to and repeat a nonsense word	
To blend the sounds of a word together and identify it from individual spoken sounds	
To identify and say the separate syllables that make up words	
To listen to an instruction and carry out actions in the right sequence as part of a group	
To listen to and respond appropriately to a word	
To identify the first sound in a word	
To listen to and copy a rhythm	
To blend and segment the sounds of a short word	
To listen to and respond appropriately to a sound	
To say the two sounds in a nonsense word	
To identify the last sound in a word	
To listen to and follow an instruction	
To identify the middle sound in a word	
Date:	**Child's name:**

Starting the programme

Routledge
Taylor & Francis Group

Set-up meeting agenda

At:

On:

Present:

Speech and language therapist/Specialist teacher

Inclusion coordinator

Reception class teacher

Classroom assistant(s)

Topics	Resources
Identified staff to deliver group sessions and contact arrangements • Speech and language therapist • Reception class teacher • Classroom assistant(s)	
Service Description Discuss queries	Service Description
Service Agreement To be drawn up and signed if the service is to be jointly delivered in collaboration with an external form of SEN support, eg NHS speech and language therapist	Service Agreement
Timetable for groups Agree and complete a timetable sheet Agree a designated room in which the groups may meet	Timetable sheet
Resources Agree when and who will make, and keep, resources	Printer, laminator, storage system Time to make up the set of resources
School policy for informing parents and carers	Handout for parents
Signs and symbols Consider linking *School Start* to the existing use of signing systems or agree to begin using signing systems (such as Makaton, *Cued Articulation* and *Jolly Phonics*)	

(continued)

Topics	Resources
Achieving liaison between staff through the year to promote transfer of skills into the classroom and home Classroom assistant(s) and class teacher/home	
Sharing case history information (For example, with local speech and language therapy department)	
End-of-year evaluation process Agree who will assess the progress of children, using the checklist	
Other training requirements For example, in Makaton	
Date for *School Start* training session	

183

Training meeting agenda

At:

On:

Present:

Speech and language therapist/

Inclusion coordinator

Reception class teacher

Classroom assistant(s)

Topics	Resources
Using the checklists At the beginning and end of *School Start*	Language Sessions Checklist Sound Awareness Sessions Checklist
Setting activities from the checklist For the classroom or home. The activities have been written so that they can also be used as educational targets	Resource Templates are available at www.routledge.com/cw/speechmark
Resources Discuss using real objects where possible, preparing picture resources and linking in with the use of signs and symbol systems	Resource Templates are available at www.routledge.com/cw/speechmark
How to run groups Discuss the principles of successful groups (for example, gelling games)	'Tips for running the Language and Sound Awareness Sessions' handouts
Looking at the programme Learning objectives (linked to the Foundation Stage Curriculum) Group Session Sheets Note keeping and records of completed: • Checklists • Group Session Sheets • Child Evaluation Records	*School Start*
Working with support services Discuss working as a team within the school, and liaison with support services, including the local speech and language therapy service	Resource Templates are available at www.routledge.com/cw/speechmark

(continued)

Topics	Resources
Collaborative working as a team What the class teacher needs to know from the SLT or classroom assistant What the classroom assistant needs to know from the SLT or class teacher What the SLT needs to know from the class teacher or classroom assistant For example: substituting vocabulary from the classroom; giving the class teacher objectives for the six-week block; sending parents copies of their child's evaluation record; revising classroom targets for the child at the end of each term	'Handout for Home and Class' (one for each six-week block)
Suggestions for further reading and training	*Teaching Children with Speech and Language Difficulties* (Martin, 2000)

School Start Language and Sound Awareness Groups

Notes for parents

The school is pleased to be able to offer a targeted group intervention to develop the language and communication skills of identified children in reception class. Classroom assistants will follow a set programme written by speech and language therapists: the *School Start* programme. This consists of communication games played in a small group throughout Reception year. The games are designed to improve skills for listening, talking and literacy. The games are also linked to the Early Years Foundation Stage early learning goals.

The school will monitor how your child achieves the learning objectives at the end of each six-week block of sessions. To help your child use these new skills outside the group, you may be given a handout summarising what your child has learned with ideas on how you may support these by playing communication games at home.

The reception class teacher will monitor the children's progress over the year. This will contribute towards the Early Years Foundation Stage Profile, which is completed for every child at the end of the Reception year.

We hope that you will welcome this opportunity for your child to be included in this communication programme. If you have any further queries, please arrange to speak to your child's reception class teacher.

Tips for running the Language Sessions

- Include up to six children in the group, selected using the checklist.

- Each session to last 20–30 minutes.

- Allow 5–10 minutes before the session to prepare the room and materials and review the activities.

- Allow 5–10 minutes after the session to tidy up, mark the Group Session Sheet and give feedback to the class teacher.

- Keep the time slot and the room for the group constant wherever possible.

- Liaise with the class teacher; use the 'Handout for Home and Class' for each six-week block of sessions to identify the topic vocabulary being used within the classroom. You may substitute some vocabulary in the activities with that currently being taught in class.

- Give Home Sheets to parents so that they can reinforce the vocabulary and concepts covered in the sessions; send home the appropriate 'Handout for Home and Class'.

- At the end of each six-week block, complete the Child Evaluation Record; give copies of this to the class teacher and the parents.

- Remember: praise positive behaviours
  ignore negative behaviours
  make group rules clear and keep to them
  make the aim of each activity explicit
  seat the children in a semi-circle
  minimise potential distractions.

This is a play-based intervention; find ways to get the children moving and doing under adult guidance and structure.

Tips for running the Sound Awareness Sessions

- Include up to six children in the group, selected using the checklist.

- Each session to last 20–30 minutes.

- Allow 5–10 minutes before the session to prepare the room and materials and review the activities.

- Allow 5–10 minutes after the session to tidy up, mark the Group Session Sheet and give feedback to the class teacher.

- Keep the time slot and the room for the group constant wherever possible.

- Give the class teacher a copy of the 'Handout for Home and Class' at the start of each six-week block of sessions.

- At the end of each six-week block, complete the Child Evaluation Record; give copies of this to the class teacher and the parents.

- Remember: praise positive behaviours
  ignore negative behaviours
  make group rules clear and keep to them
  make the aim of each activity explicit
  seat the children in a semi-circle
  minimise potential distractions.

This is a play-based intervention; find ways to get the children moving and doing under adult guidance and structure.

Signs and symbols list

You will find it useful to learn the signs and use the symbols for the words listed below. Your local speech and language therapy department will be able to advise you on how to obtain training and support in an appropriate sign and symbol system, such as Makaton®.

above	her	not fruit	she
and	here	not furniture	slow
behind	him	not metal	there
below	his	not paper	top
big	I	not plastic	toy
bigger	in	not toy	tree
body	in front	not vegetables	under
bottom	last	not wood	vegetables
clothes	light	on	what?
different	little	paper	where?
empty	many	plant	who?
first	metal	plastic	wood
fruit	middle	pull	yes
full	mine	push	you
furniture	my	quick	your
go	next	sad	yours
happy	no	same	
he	not	shapes	

Handouts for home and class

School Start

Sample Service Agreement and Description

Your school is being offered the opportunity to join together with

_____ (insert name of service)

to bring a programme of Language and Sound Awareness Group Sessions to your children in Reception year.

The *School Start* programme is designed to continue throughout the entire year and will involve:

- identifying and assessing appropriate children
- training for reception class staff
- setting classroom targets and implementing classroom strategies.

A speech and language therapist (SLT) or specialist teacher in conjunction with school-provided classroom assistants will deliver the programme to two groups, focusing separately on:

- Language
- Sound Awareness.

The aims of *School Start* are to:

- develop the language and communication skills of identified children in the Reception year, using a preventive approach by tackling difficulties in early years and to supplement other local speech and language services
- train schools to sustain a rolling programme of Language and Sound Awareness Groups for reception-age children
- provide an easy-to-follow Language and Sound Awareness programme, linked to the Foundation Stage Curriculum which classroom assistants find easy to deliver.

Please read the following service description and discuss any queries with:

_____ (insert contact details)

If you wish to proceed, please return a signed copy of the service agreement.

Service Description

First six weeks of the reception year

Set-up

- The *School Start* service agreement is discussed and signed.
- The school identifies staff who will deliver the sessions in conjunction with the local speech and language therapists (SLTs) or specialist teachers.
- Dates are agreed with the school for training and timetables for group delivery.

Training of reception class staff

The reception class teacher and classroom assistants meet the SLT for one hour's training on identification or assessment and the programme. It is recommended that the inclusion coordinator (INCo) also attends the training in order to oversee the process.

Identifying and assessing appropriate children

The reception teacher uses initial observations of the children, together with knowledge of any history of speech and language delay, to identify children who may benefit from the *School Start* programme, for example, children who have been previously referred to speech and language therapy.

The relevant checklist is completed for the children identified.

A final list of up to six children is selected for each of the two groups (Language and Sound Awareness). Some children may attend both groups. The composition of the groups will remain constant throughout the year, except in exceptional circumstances agreed with the SLT.

Signs and symbols

School Start is designed to be used in conjunction with signs and symbols for concepts (such as Makaton) and speech sounds (such as *Cued Articulation* or *Jolly Phonics*) – see the following references.

References

Lloyd S (1995) *The Jolly Phonics Starter Kit*, Jolly Learning Ltd, Chigwell (www.jollylearning.co.uk).

Passey J (1985) *Cued Articulation*, Stass Publications, Ponteland (www.stasspublications.co.uk).

Walker M & Ferris-Taylor R (1998) *Parent/Carer Training Pack 1 & Pack 2*, Makaton Vocabulary Development Project, Camberley (www.makaton.org).

Programme delivery during reception year

Setting classroom targets and implementing strategies

- The completed checklist is used to identify individual classroom targets and activities for home using the appropriate handouts – 'Suggested activities for the classroom and home'.

- Once *School Start* begins, it is strongly recommended that there is close liaison between the staff running the groups and the class teacher. This will ensure that there is continuity between the group activities and the classroom activities for the transference of newly acquired skills.

- The class teacher may also require time to consult with the SLT to ensure good communication in the classroom; the class teacher will raise this need directly with the SLT.

The *School Start* programme

- The programme contains the aims, required resources and activities for each group programme.

- The templates can be photocopied, and colour templates are available at www.routledge.com/cw/speechmark

- To support and train the delivery of the programme, the SLT will co-deliver an agreed number of sessions as follows: (please complete)

- The school will deliver all 30 *School Start* sessions between October and July

Evaluation of progress – July

- The school readministers the relevant checklist for each child.

- The checklist data from the beginning and end of *School Start* will be assembled for analysis by the school/SLT (delete as appropriate).

- Results from the July checklist may be used to identify appropriate targets and strategies for Year 1.

The school commitment

- To provide at least one classroom assistant (preferably two) to deliver the two groups throughout the Reception year.
- To timetable two 50-minute slots (30–40 minutes' delivery and approximately 15 minutes' preparation time) weekly for the groups, in negotiation with the SLT.
- The reception class teaching staff will assess the children using the relevant checklists at the beginning and end of *School Start*.
- The INCo will oversee the delivery of the programme.
- The reception teacher and classroom assistants will be available to meet with the SLT for training.
- The school will provide a suitable room in which the sessions can take place.
- The school will provide the resources needed for the activities (these are materials commonly found in school, including scissors and paper).
- To provide replacement classroom assistant(s) should staff leave during the school year.
- To inform the SLT as soon as possible should an appointment need to be cancelled (for example, if the children or classroom assistants are not in school).
- To give the SLT prior notice should the class teacher wish to discuss an individual child on the programme.

Confirmation of agreement

Return to _____ (insert service name)

I wish to access this service and have read the above information:

Signed: _____

For: _____ (school name)

Date: _____

Handout for Home and Class: Language Sessions Weeks 1–6

Learning objectives

- To work as part of a group, taking turns and sharing
- To sustain attentive listening
- To follow rules in a group
- To match two pictures that are the same
- To investigate objects and materials using all of their senses
- To find named items on request (toy animals or other toys, 'big', 'little', Christmas vocabulary)
- To extend word knowledge (understand and use the concept 'same' and the pronoun 'I', 'a' before an item and 'yes'/'no')

Summary of vocabulary, concepts and syntax

Vocabulary	Concepts	Syntax	Other skills
• children's names	• same	• pronoun 'I'	• taking turns
• classroom objects	• yes/no	• article 'a'	• listening and waiting for a word
• animals	• big/little		• good sitting
• Christmas			• making eye contact
• food			

Suggested activities for home and class

To sort objects into two categories, big and little

Start by showing the child 'big' and 'not big' objects. Demonstrate 'sitting on the "big" chair', 'sitting on the "not big" chair'. Using toy and real-size matching objects, get the child to follow instructions using 'big' and 'not big'. When this has been achieved, introduce 'little' in contrast with 'big'. Consolidate with a variety of objects and picture materials.

To choose one toy from a choice of two and play with it for two minutes

Control and limit the available toys. Remove distractions. Comment on the child's actions as he plays, for example: 'Jack is blowing the trumpet'.

Handout for Home and Class: Language Sessions Weeks 7–12

Learning objectives

- To arrange items into categories
- To find named items on request (body parts and kitchenware)
- To find and name an item on request (clothes)
- To understand and use the concepts 'first', 'last' and 'different'
- To investigate objects and materials using touch
- To understand the prepositions 'on', 'in', 'under'
- To extend word knowledge (understand and use 'what', 'and', 'my', 'mine', 'your', 'you' and regular plural forms, such as 'book'/'books')

Summary of vocabulary, concepts and syntax

Vocabulary	Concepts	Syntax	Other skills
• furniture	• on	• and	• taking turns
• food	• different	• what	• using touch
• body parts	• in	• my	
• kitchenware	• first	• mine	
• toys	• under	• your, you	
• clothes	• last	• regular plurals	

Suggested activities for home and class

To name 10 familiar items found in a classroom or at home

Begin by checking that the child can understand the vocabulary: for example, check that he can pick up the item from a selection on request. Devise a game so that the child picks up an object and gives it to another child, naming the object (for example, shopping games). Set up situations where the child has to ask an adult for the equipment they need for a task.

To sustain play with a chosen toy for five minutes

Allow the child to choose from two favoured activities. Remove all other toys and distractions. Support and praise the child for refocusing on the activity. Build up to five minutes' play with one toy. Help the child to complete the activity: for example, do the first half of the jigsaw puzzle for him.

Handout for Home and Class: Language Sessions Weeks 13–18

Learning objectives

- To find named items on request (parts of a house)
- To find and name an item on request (light sources)
- To understand and use the concepts 'big', 'bigger', 'middle' and 'little' in relation to size, the prepositions 'behind' and 'in front of', and the adjectives 'quick' and 'slow'
- To extend word knowledge (understand and use the words 'he' and 'she', regular plurals, 'his' and 'her', 'and' to link two verbs, and 'no' with a noun)
- To arrange items into categories according to the materials that they are made from
- To ask a question using 'Who?' and 'Where?'

Summary of vocabulary, concepts and syntax

Vocabulary	Concepts	Syntax	Other skills
• parts of a house	• big	• he	• listening
• light sources	• little	• she	• taking turns
• wood items	• middle-sized	• singular	
• metal items	• bigger	• plural	
• fruit	• wood/not wood	• his	
• plastic	• metal/not metal	• her	
	• in front	• 'and' with verbs	
	• behind	• who	
	• quick	• where	
	• slow	• 'no' with a noun	

Suggested activities for home and class

To put a toy 'on' the table; to put a toy 'under' the chair

Teach one instruction first in a variety of settings. Gradually reduce non-verbal cues until the child is following the verbal instruction alone. Use picture materials and ask the child to point to something in the picture using the target words. Extend the activity by using instructions containing 'above' and 'below'.

To sort bricks or pencils into three colour groups and to name the colour groups

You will need bricks or pencils of three colours – red, green and blue – and three boxes. Show the child how to sort the bricks or pencils into the boxes according to colour. Check that they can do this activity without help.

For the next step you will need only two boxes. Put the blue bricks or pencils into one box, saying the word 'blue' as you put them into the box. Then put the other colour bricks or pencils into the other box, saying the words 'not blue' as you put the remaining bricks or pencils into the box. Ask the child to repeat the activity after you.

When the child is successful with this task, repeat sorting the objects into 'red' and 'not red', and 'green' and 'not green'. Children benefit from having at least one day's break before moving on to a new colour label.

Handout for Home and Class: Language Sessions Weeks 9–24

Learning objectives

- To arrange items into categories (materials that they are made from, 'vegetables and 'not vegetables')
- To understand and use the concepts 'above', 'below', 'top', 'bottom', 'full', 'empty', 'push', 'pull'
- To extend word knowledge: asking 'What is it?', 'Is it …?'; understanding the pronouns 'him', 'her', 'yours'; using 'an' before a noun beginning with a vowel; saying 'It is' when describing something
- To find named items on request (tools, shapes, toy baby animals)
- To investigate objects and materials using touch (tools and shapes)
- To sustain attentive listening
- To name items (in relation to baby animals)

Summary of vocabulary, concepts and syntax

Vocabulary	Concepts	Syntax	Other skills
• vegetables	• above	• what?	• listening
• tools	• below	• is it?	• taking turns
• baby animals	• top	• it is	
• shapes	• bottom	• him	
• animals	• empty	• her	
	• full	• yours	
	• push	• an	
	• pull		
	• made of paper		
	• not made of paper		

Suggested activities for home and class

To listen to an instruction containing one action verb and to follow the instruction

The child must be able to understand without visual demonstration or reliance on context; do not, for example, show them the scissors and then ask them to cut. It is easier to do this activity in the hall or playground. The instructions can be extended to involve prepositions or adverbs (eg 'jump over', 'walk in front of me', 'run softly').

To end an activity, with preparation, and start a new activity

Show the child the two activities he will be doing. Let him choose the activity he wishes to do first. Warn the child that the first activity will end in one minute. Take away the first activity and show the child the second one. Warn the child that the second activity will end in one minute.

Handout for Home and Class: Language Sessions Weeks 25–30

Learning objectives

- To find and name an item on request (things at the farm and the seaside, parts of a tree and a plant, clothes for a hot day)
- To perform two actions in order ('first …, then …')
- To identify items within a given category
- To extend word knowledge (understand 'happy', 'sad', 'many' and ask 'Who?')
- To remember two items after a short time delay
- To name an item when given a description
- To use the structure 'It is not' in sentences
- To understand vocabulary related to body parts
- To understand and use the terms 'here', 'there' and 'or'

Summary of vocabulary, concepts and syntax

Vocabulary	Concepts	Syntax	Other skills
• farms	• first …	• who?	• auditory memory
• parts of a tree	• then …	• it is not	• two items after a short delay
• parts of a plant	• happy	• there	
• seaside	• sad	• here	
• clothes for a hot day	• many	• or	
• body parts			

Suggested activities for home and class

To listen to a story or information and show attention through asking or answering questions or completing a follow-on activity

Check active listening for extended periods (for example, during a five-minute story) by asking questions. Ensure that the level of the language used is appropriate for the child's comprehension.

To follow instructions containing 'many', 'less' and 'bigger'

For example, 'Get me the box with many bricks in it', 'Get me the box with less in it', 'Get me the bigger book'. Use the instructions in context and demonstrate how to follow the instruction. Gradually fade out the demonstrations.

To give five words from a category

Select a category from a known area for the child, including topic work (eg farm animals, vehicles, items you find at the post office). Use a clock or timer as the child gets more confident, to speed up responses. Keep reinforcing the concept of a category by saying, 'Yes, they are all types of …'. Reinforce by continuing to ask the child to sort objects, or pictures of objects, into categories.

Handout for Home and Class: Sound Awareness Sessions Weeks 1–6

Learning objectives

- To listen for a word and respond appropriately
- To identify noises and sounds in the environment
- To join in with a familiar nursery rhyme
- To identify which musical instrument is played from a choice of two
- To understand the concept 'first'
- To understand the concept 'last'
- To listen for a sound and respond appropriately
- To be aware of words that rhyme

Summary of concepts and skills

Concepts	Skills
• same	• listening for 'go'
• first	• listening for a target sound
• last	• rhyme judgement
• next	• auditory memory
	• taking turns

Suggested activities for home and class

To walk three steps, using 'stepping stones', saying one word of a phrase or sentence per stone

For example, the phrase might be 'cats and dogs'. The stepping stones can be made from pieces of paper in a line on the floor. Start with two-word phrases, for example 'dog barks'. Use single-syllable words. Build up to using the little grammatical words (for example, 'the' and 'is').

To identify the child who is first and last in a line at the door

Demonstrate 'first' and 'last' in real-life situations. Take one concept word at a time. Reinforce whenever possible during the day. For example, 'Put up your hand if you are first in the line. Put up your hand if you are last in the line.' Once the concepts have been learned in these situations, see if the child can talk about a picture (for example, a picture of people queuing for a bus).

Handout for Home and Class: Sound Awareness Sessions Weeks 7–12

Learning objectives

- To listen for a sound from a choice of two and respond appropriately
- To identify which words rhyme
- To understand the concept and label for 'last', 'word' and 'middle'
- To listen for a sound and respond appropriately
- To correctly identify the named word from two that sound similar
- To give an example of a word that rhymes
- To move a counter for each word

Summary of concepts and skills

Concepts	Skills
• last	• listening for individual words
• middle	• auditory discrimination of minimal pairs
• first	• rhyme judgement and generation
• next	• auditory memory
• word	• taking turns

Suggested activities for home and class

To clap out the syllables in their name and their friend's name

Demonstrate clapping a child's name and ask how many claps the children heard. Ask each child to clap the syllables of their name – first with you and then independently.

To have speech that is clearly understood by unfamiliar adults

When the child says a word incorrectly, use the technique known as 'modelling'. This means that you repeat the word clearly for the child to hear but do not put on any pressure for the child to repeat it. If the child does attempt to repeat the word after you, praise them for the effort ('Good try!'). You can play games that encourage the child to hear the difference between the word said correctly and incorrectly (for example, 'Give me the cat' versus 'Give me the tat').

Handout for Home and Class: Sound Awareness Sessions Weeks 13–18

Learning objectives

- To listen carefully to other people
- To identify which words rhyme
- To move a counter for each word
- To listen for a word in a story
- To give examples of words that rhyme
- To identify the first, middle and last words from a list of three
- To identify the first, middle and last words from a phrase

Summary of concepts and skills

Concepts	Skills
• last	• sentence repetition
• middle	• listening for an embedded target word
• first	• rhyme judgement and generation
• next	• auditory memory
• word	• phoneme substitution
	• taking turns

Suggested activities for home and class

To pick up two pictures of objects which have names that rhyme, from a choice of three

Put down three pictures and name each picture for the child. Then ask the child to give you the two that rhyme. The child may find the task easier with toy objects than pictures. The child may need a visual reminder to listen to the 'end' of the word: for example, you could show him a picture of a train with carriages, and put a brick on the 'end' carriage.

To collect three items in the classroom, the playground or the home

Ask the child to collect the three named items. Encourage the child to repeat the list, using his fingers as he says each item, before carrying out the activity. Extend by using objects that are further away so that the instruction has to be retained for longer periods of time. Use in game situations, such as 'shopping'.

Routledge
Taylor & Francis Group
203

Handout for Home and Class: Sound Awareness Sessions Weeks 19–24

Learning objectives

- To identify familiar sounds
- To give examples of words that rhyme
- To move a counter for each word
- To listen for a word and respond appropriately
- To identify and say the separate syllables that make up words
- To listen for a sound and respond appropriately
- To listen to and follow an instruction
- To listen for a sound in a word and respond appropriately

Summary of concepts and skills

Concepts	Skills
• last	• phoneme substitution
• middle	• auditory discrimination of words or sounds
• first	• rhyme judgement and generation
• next	• auditory memory
	• syllable identification and segmentation
	• taking turns

Suggested activities for home and class

To listen to two spoken words and say whether they do or do not rhyme

Start with easy examples. For instance, you might use the child's name: 'Thomas, pie', 'pie, sky'. Refer back to the train picture and praise the child for listening to the ends of the words.

To go to another adult and deliver a short verbal message

Use familiar adults and a known route, for example the route to the office if in school. Give the children a written back-up in case they forget the message (the other adult can use this to prompt them if they forget part of the message). Make the child repeat the message back to you two times before they go.

Handout for Home and Class: Sound Awareness Sessions Weeks 25–30

Learning objectives

- To listen to and repeat a nonsense word
- To blend the sounds of a word together and identify the word from individual spoken sounds
- To identify and say the separate syllables that make up words
- To listen to an instruction and carry out actions in the right sequence as part of a group
- To listen to and respond appropriately to a word
- To identify the first sound in a word
- To listen to and copy a rhythm
- To blend and segment the sounds of a short word
- To listen to and respond appropriately to a sound
- To say the two sounds in a nonsense word
- To identify the last sound in a word
- To listen to and follow an instruction
- To identify the middle sound in a word

Summary of concepts and skills

Concepts	Skills
• last	• phoneme identification, substitution and blending
• middle	• auditory discrimination of words or sounds
• first	• rhythm
• next	• auditory memory
	• syllable identification, segmentation and blending
	• taking turns

Suggested activities for home and class

To listen to two sounds and blend to say the word

Start with blending syllables: for example, 'mu' + 'mee' = 'mummy'. Move on to simple words that have two sounds (for example, 'car', 'key'). Use the actual sounds; for example, make sure that 's' does not have 'uh' on the end when you say it in isolation. Use *Cued Articulation* (Passey, 1985a, 1985b) if you know it. Say the syllables or sounds with minimal intonation. If the child is able, move on to words with three sounds (for example, 'cup', 'rock').

To have speech that is clearly understood by unfamiliar adults

When the child says a word incorrectly, use the technique known as 'modelling'. This means that you repeat the word clearly for the child to hear but do not put on any pressure for the child to repeat it. If the child does attempt to repeat the word after you, praise them for the effort ('Good try!'). You can play games that encourage the child to hear the difference between the word said correctly and incorrectly (for example, 'Give me the cat' versus 'Give me the tat').

Bibliography

Department for Education and Skills (DfES) (2004) *Every Child Matters: Change for Children*, DfES, London.

Gascoigne M (2015) *The Balanced System*, online, www.mgaconsulting.org.uk/who-we-are/marie-gascoigne/ (accessed May 2015).

Lloyd S (1995a) *The Jolly Phonics Starter Kit*, Jolly Learning Ltd, Chigwell (www.jollylearning.co.uk).

Lloyd S (1995b) *The Phonics Handbook*, Jolly Learning Ltd, Chigwell (www.jollylearning.co.uk).

Martin D (2000) *Teaching Children with Speech and Language Difficulties*, David Fulton Publishers/ Routledge, London.

Marvin C (1990) 'Problems in school-based language and collaboration services', *Language, Speech and Hearing Services in Schools*, 25, pp258–68.

Passey J (1985a) *Cued Articulation*, Stass Publications, Ponteland (www.stasspublications.co.uk).

Passey J (1985b) *Cued Articulation Charts*, Stass Publications, Ponteland (www.stasspublications.co.uk).

Passey J (1985c) *Cued Vowels*, Stass Publications, Ponteland (www.stasspublications.co.uk).

Passey J (2000) *Seeing a Sound* (video), Stass Publications, Ponteland (www.stasspublications.co.uk).

UK Government (2014a) *The Code of Practice*, online, www.gov.uk/.../data/.../SEND_Code_of_ Practice_January_2015.pdf (accessed May 2015).

UK Government Standards and Testing Agency (2014b) *Exemplification of EYFS Profile*, online, www.gov.uk/government/publications/early-years-foundation-stage-profile-handbook/exemplification-of-eyfs-profile-expected-descriptors (accessed May 2015).

Walker M & Ferris-Taylor R (1998) *Parent/Carer Training Pack* for the *Makaton* Core Vocabulary Pack 1 & Pack 2, Makaton Vocabulary Development Project, Camberley (www.makaton.org).